through the inner chatter and self-doubt that keep us *all* stuck. When Cheyenne writes, 'Give yourself permission to go as big with your dreams as you do with your worries,' she's not just offering an idea . . . she'll also show you how. Cannot recommend this book enough."

—Britt Frank, LSCSW, SEP, author of
The Science of Stuck and Align Your Mind

"Yasmine has written a potent, relatable guide for reconnecting with ourselves. The actions she suggests and the questions she prompts hold a mirror up to readers and help them take steps toward the life they truly want."

—Juanita Tolliver, author of A More Perfect Party:
The Night Shirley Chisholm and Diahann Carroll
Reshaped Politics and host of Archival podcast

THE **COMEBACK** ERA

From

LIMITING

BELIEFS

to

LIVING

WITHOUT

LIMITS

THE
COMEBACK
ERA

Yasmine Cheyenne

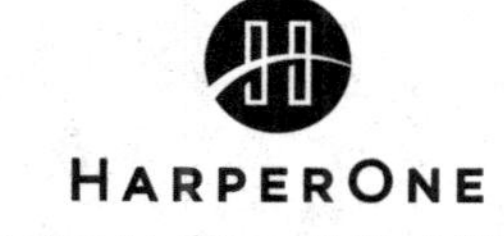

HarperOne

An Imprint of HarperCollins*Publishers*

*To my Little You: Look at how far we've come.
Here's to always remembering who we are.*

Contents

Introduction

I was about nine years old when I made myself this promise in my tiny Brooklyn apartment: Yasmine, live your life like you're destined for more.

I've had a lot of change in my life, which sometimes felt like chaos, but it was always done with absolute intention. I make mistakes, lots of them, and yet somehow, I've always known when it was time to grow, leave, or set myself free. Part of this knowing is a deep trust in my intuition. When I made this promise to myself, I didn't know what "more" was and couldn't have dreamed of some of the experiences that I've had. But when we're open, life has a funny way of surprising us with opportunities that we never imagined possible for ourselves.

If we choose to walk with wisdom rather than expectation, we open up our lives to opportunities falling right into our laps. However, most of us don't live that way because we follow a structured path, hoping it will be enough. For some of us, it's more than enough. For others, we're only living out a tiny percentage of what we're capable of.

I've always been intrigued by transformation and the work it takes to make a decision to do something different. Every ounce of us has been living life one way, and now we've decided to do something new, because either we're inspired or the Universe is. Change is beautiful, but it doesn't always arrive that way.

While writing this book, I found myself momentarily putting these pages down for my husband's résumé. He received an unsolicited invitation from the Universe, prompting a potential career change, and, of course, I was there to help. In that moment, it felt like my words were coming to life in our lives. The leadership where he worked changed, and everything he thought was safe about his job changed too. With the unknowns feeling uncomfortably close, we settled into our roles: him frozen and unclear in which direction to go next, and me ready to change it all immediately to reduce his discomfort. I have always excelled in chaos and commotion, holding it together with a *fix-it* energy. As I mentioned earlier, I move with intention, but sometimes we're asked to pause and check in rather than move. As we started to claim our "normal" roles, ready to perform, I didn't want to create from that energy. And when I shared this with my husband, he didn't either.

WE'D BEEN TALKING A LOT ABOUT HIS PURPOSE, AND we chalked it up to the research for this book. The more he thought about his purpose, the clearer he could see that he needed *more*. I noticed that his definition of "purpose" was evolving as he became more comfortable defining it beyond his work. A conscious shift took place within himself, and then, suddenly, an invitation for change appeared. When you have a secure job that provides insurance and retirement and is unlikely to go away anytime soon, changing it never feels like a smart thing to do. Without the Universe bringing potential change to him, I don't believe he would've thought about leaving. He'd known for some time this job wasn't enough, but he also knew he could do it for the next thirty years *for us*.

My husband's decision to take a job he loathed *for us* isn't different from what many of us are doing right now, and we don't only do it at work. We do it in friendships, relationships, and more. We push through because of what we feel we deserve, as well as who we think we must be to the people around us. It's about paying bills, putting food on the table, and stability. Many of us are searching for our purpose while doing what we feel we must.

While waiting to find out his job status, he practiced what I invite you to do: Reconnect with younger versions of yourself, or as I like to call it, "*Little You*." He thought about what brought him joy when he was younger, and it was always sports, specifically soccer—a sport he hadn't dedicated time to and now regretted.

Our youngest daughter was already in soccer, and I'd mentioned to him before all this change came up that I thought he would be a great coach, but he didn't sign up. Our daughter's league was short staffed, but adult responsibilities made him feel like he couldn't add one more thing. But now, with everything we had going on, I countered. "We're already at her practices. You sure you don't want to give it a try?" At the next practice, he decided to help the coach, and after it was over, he shared that he hadn't had as much fun as he did that evening in a long time. It wasn't as if the stress from his job situation disappeared, but spending time doing something that lit him up created a reconnection with himself. He signed up as a coach that evening and has felt more alive and fulfilled ever since. His younger self is leading this new journey, and it's something he thought he'd never get to do, as he believed it was *too late*. No, he wasn't playing on the team, but he was part of it, and it mattered. Seeing our dreams come true, even when they feel late, matters.

Whenever I'm about to pivot, there are always signs within and around me beforehand. The job that once felt great feels like a drag. The relationship that I had hoped would improve now feels suffocating. My morning energy is traded for lethargy. The intensity of these signs becomes more ferocious the longer we ignore our inner knowing.

What I'm sure you've noticed, if you've been silently craving change, is that your lack of contentment extends far beyond your job. You may have an excellent partner or kids and still feel like something is missing. You may have the job you worked so hard for and wonder if you even want it anymore. Sometimes, *something is missing*; **we do need more**. And other times, what we're looking for is a sense of grounded satiety in who we are, which can't come from anything other than a deep sense of peace. A peace defined by meeting life's moments with grace, laughter, disbelief, or rage. In other words, being so content in who we are and where we are in the moment that we know our peace can't only mean calm seas. Instead, the waves can rise and crash against each other, bringing peace too. If the ocean isn't peace and surrender, then what is?

The nagging feeling that visits and says *this isn't enough for you anymore* will remind you what once felt fresh and new has now become dormant, and there's an invitation for change. For some, the invitation will be toward the thing you've been ignoring that you've always known mattered to you. For others, the call will be toward something you never imagined possible. Some will initiate the change on their own, while others get dragged into a transformation they weren't ready for. However change finds you, almost all of us can pinpoint the moment that made us finally say yes, when we'd said no so many times before.

The journey we're taking has three parts and many invitations. You'll find invitations for growth, stretching you beyond what you've allowed in the past. An invitation to finally answer the ache you feel when your feet hit the floor in the morning, and you know you're about to spend more time doing what everyone else expects of you rather than what you desire. The journey will be led in part by Little You, the younger version of yourself that many of us have tried to please by attempting to adult "the right way" rather than reconnecting with who we are. You'll be reminded of the promises you made to Little You; promises that feel so far away, they're whispers now. But this is an invitation to stop the cycle of your life that feels like rinse and repeat and get excited enough to *want to* dream again.

You might notice that life tried to get your attention before, and you only have the clarity to see this now because you've finally said yes. Just because you didn't answer life's knocks on your door in the past doesn't mean this is an invitation to berate yourself. Having your awareness back is a moment for gratitude because, despite all the noise, **you heard the call this time, and you listened.** Accept the invitation, knowing that for whatever reason, today you are a yes. You can open it when you're ready, and know the invite may be more of a feeling than words. Sometimes it's a dream, it might come as a memory, and when you receive words, they may come from the person you least expected. No one else's beliefs, explanations, expectations, or desires get to reside here. This time, this invitation is for you.

I don't know if life imitates art or if art imitates life, but I know that everything I'm sharing in this book, I've lived through. Even though I'd promised myself I'd always pivot when necessary, especially when it was hard, uncomfortable, or scary, I know firsthand the awkward journey of coming back to yourself because I've been there. It's important, to most, to have someone guiding you who knows this is the most uncomfortable work to commit to. It's not easy, yet it's changed my life. And beyond me, each wonderful person I interviewed who shares their truth throughout these pages has put into words what I, my clients, and the random Uber drivers who've turned our cab rides into confessionals have admitted they feel. There *has* to be more to life than this.

I will share the stories of amazing women: Lia, Britt, Deesha, Chloe, and Amanda. These women have left me in awe as they've navigated their brave journeys and are still taking small step after small step, building a life and world for themselves that is beautiful. I hope you realize, through their stories, that what you're navigating isn't new, and I hope it brings calm energy to your nervous system to know someone has made it through to the other side of what you're trying to get through. I hope their stories are an affirmation that you can make it through too.

And ultimately, I hope by looking at your own story, through curious eyes, you remember you've always found a way. You've always found the light.

Allow any previously closed or dormant places to reopen.

Allow life to surprise you with opportunities you never believed possible.

Rekindle the fire that has gone out.

I'll tell you just as I told my nine-year-old self: Live your life like you're destined for more.

And say yes to coming back home to you.

PART I

Curiosity

I READ THIS QUOTE BY EMILY DICKINSON. "I'm out with lanterns, looking for myself." And I immediately felt the ache and desperation to know ourselves, and to try, however we can, to find ourselves again. Emily doesn't mention this, but I presume that if you're holding a lantern, the looking, the searching, is happening in the dark, when you can't see clearly. It's brave to reunite with the real us by remembering the part of ourselves we feel we've lost.

It's also the definition of living a curious life and being willing to search, to find, to know.

I'm the kind of person who is also out at night, with lanterns, looking for others. I often wonder, *Did you experience this too? Are you searching too? Is there someone else out there who's been through this too?* Being allowed to hear people's stories is an incredible honor. I love knowing how you became you.

Each woman in this book graciously agreed to share their story with me, with us, and to be honest, without a lot of convincing or details. I've sprinkled pieces of their stories throughout, and they've become powerful reminders that through others' stories, we reclaim our hope. Through their perseverance, we find our strength. And through their searching, we see ourselves.

Take in these words and let them awaken you when you're ready.

To searching.

1
What Did Little You Always Know Was True?

There comes a point in our adult lives when fun feels optional. Everything is so serious. Everything is *I have to*. Everything feels unbelievably too much. The pendulum dramatically swings from more play than work to all work, no play, and it shows. We see the sunrise, not because we've been out all night laughing and dancing until daybreak, but because we get up at that hour to get through the amount of *stuff* happening daily.

We are tired. We are cynical. We are overworked and we under play. We are hardworking and often without reward. We are pretending to be okay through dinners, through friend meetups, and at kid pickup. We laugh through our dissatisfaction, making jokes through our frozen smiles, a representation of how chillingly odd our lives feel.

Somewhere down the line, we were yanked into lives we barely recognize. How did all our hard work, all our promises to do it differently than our parents, all our dreams to partner differently, all our vows to never lose ourselves, all our whispers to our friends at dinners to always stay close . . . turn into this? Lives that we preface with those famous words, "I **mean . . . I can't really complain, right?**"

Can you "not really" complain, or do you believe there's nothing you can do?

When did what you were working for in your relationships, in your career, in every area of your life, become lost? When did you seemingly lose your sense of purpose?

This is the time when older age feels closer than youth, and we get a flurry of brilliant ideas. We think, *well, if I'm lost, let's get found.*

Insert: *the crisis.*

Whether you experience yours at twenty-five, forty, after kids, after marriage, or all of the above, societally we recognize these periods of rebellion as counter to the significant transformation that took place in our lives and changed the foundation of who we thought we were, *even if we wanted the change that occurred.*

Of course, *you want to get older.* But it doesn't make the changes and the reality of mortality being closer than it's ever been any easier. It doesn't make the fact that there's still so much you want to do, but haven't, any easier, especially when you're struggling to figure out who you are and what it's all for. I think we're all trying to figure out *what it's all for.*

And because the transformation from twenty to thirty to forty and beyond feels like a face slap that came out of nowhere, as you grow older, you're probably thinking more carefully about what you say yes to. Spending our time now feels like spending a thousand dollars. We run through a list of questions, fine-tooth comb–style, before we commit to anything. For a lot of us, this *careful commitment ritual* keeps us doing pretty much nothing at all. Again, we don't say yes until we understand *what it's all for.*

In the same breath, things that used to feel like something we'd never get to do now feel nonnegotiable. This now seems like the perfect time to get the motorcycle. The perfect time to dye your hair pink. The perfect time to get the divorce you knew you needed ten years ago. It's the perfect time, because you know you can't ignore time. It has, as they say, caught up. You're desperate for change and go after it with full speed.

I question the notion that we experience a *midlife crisis*. It was never a crisis. It's more of a wake-up call. It's a midlife redirection. It's not a *midlife crisis,* it's **midlife clarity**. It's not a *midlife crisis;* it's a **midlife comeback.**

This period is an invitation to reconnect with what Little You always knew to be true about you. You're attempting to embrace all that you're capable of, and not in the sense of what you can *do*. The love, the connection, the peace, the joy, and the freedom too. It's an invitation back to curiosity, when you explored as a way of being. It's an invitation toward your purpose. *Your unique purpose and what you bring to the world is what it's all for.*

But why is reconnecting to what you know to be true so hard? And how did you get sidetracked in the first place?

Let's remember where we came from: The people who swaddled you in soft blankets, slathered your face with Vaseline to keep the cold air from penetrating your precious skin, or the people who did the very bare minimum but were still all you had; we come from the folks who raised us. Their opinions, their thinking-out-loud moments, and their beliefs. They all landed deeply within you. And whether they convinced you to go for "it" or convinced you to choose a safer route, they convinced you to do something.

Every single person I spoke with in the interviews mentioned *societal beliefs* as a reason they said yes to something that **wasn't** for them. And I'm sure you can think of times in your life when the "yes" that escaped your lips, a "yes" you believed was a key unlocking your life ahead, turned out instead to be a key to the cage you'd feel trapped in later. But hindsight is something we only experience over time. Our curiosity is the portal to freeing us. No keys are needed.

If I had to express who Lia was using one word, it would be "curious." She listens like no one I've ever met, letting each word land with the same importance. Nothing is insignificant when you're talking to her, and it's as if she knows that each sentence you're sharing with her has been dying to come out. Of course, she is also a brilliant therapist, and it's not surprising that she brings that same care wherever she goes, because she brings all the important things with her everywhere. She's all heart in the best way.

When talking to Lia, I asked:

You mentioned knowing you could handle holding space for adults as a child, which was a big task for Little You. Did little Lia know she wanted to be a therapist? What did she want to be when she grew up?

Lia: There was an inner knowing, and then there was the hiding of the inner knowing. My dad grew up with a lot of shame for not being educated or successful in a way that was defined here in the US. He would wear a Harvard hat and a Harvard shirt, but he didn't go to Harvard. He didn't go to college. And I then was like, "Oh, I should want to go to Harvard." And I learned about what neuroscience was. And I was like, "That sounds like a smart career." And so, I would tell people I want to be a neuroscientist. But underneath that, I really wanted to be a writer. And amid a lot of the ups and downs of my childhood, the page was where I was able to tell the truth.

Get Curious

Reflect for a moment: Were there times in your life, especially when you were younger, when you knew that what you wanted conflicted with what was expected of you? What inner knowing may have been ignored by trying to fulfill others' dreams for you? Please take note of those dreams so you can make space to reclaim them.

When we were little, we aligned with *doing the right thing* by following the advice of the people raising us. We wanted to meet their gaze, looking exactly like the dream they imagined, and for many, that meant we didn't think what we wanted had a place. Some of us heard that our desires didn't matter explicitly, and some of us internalized it without anyone telling us that who we are wasn't gonna be enough. But the burying of our truth began. The hiding began.

When I guide people through inner-child work, the mere

image of who they were as a kid can bring tears. The bright light within them, the freedom, the hopes, the mistakes not yet made, all the things we've been trying to give that part of ourselves all these years show up now. But Little You shouldn't have had to work hard to matter. Little You should've just mattered: your thoughts, your beliefs, every part of you.

> ### Get Curious
>
> When you think about Little You, what age immediately comes to mind? Are you six or sixteen years old? Are you experiencing something limiting or tough at this age, or are you at the peak of joy? Is it hard to look at Little You, or do you never want to leave this image of you?

While writing this book, I asked for childhood photos that I hadn't seen in a long time. I wanted to remember what my room looked like, what toys I played with, and how wide my smile was. I kept copies of them on my phone, so I could look at Little Yas all the time, remembering how big I was willing to dream and how much I believed in possibility. Please keep your Little You close as you read. Allow Little You's curiosity to lead you. Let Little You be excited as your head hits the pillow each night, anticipating what the next day will bring. Let them be positive, where you usually only see problems. Invite them to connect again.

Why?

Our smaller selves knew what we truly wanted. Even without all the knowledge of how we'd get what we desired, we didn't allow rules or reason to keep us from saying it out loud. It wasn't until we learned that speaking your truth isn't always a welcome conversation that our dreams went quiet. If you didn't have to abide by the rules of the world that were created for you, what would you say yes to? What would be true?

If you led your life, raised your kids, built your relationships and friendships all with the thought process of what you've always wanted, what would those things be? And more important, why is there a part of you that believes it isn't possible for you anymore? Even if the way it turns out is different from what you hoped, is it still possible?

Would you paint? Would you sail? Would you write? Would you run? Would you curate special parties, or sew?

What would you say out loud that you no longer have to hide from anyone?

The beauty of being a grown-up is that you have autonomy now. However, that doesn't make it any easier to say yes. We're still afraid that choosing ourselves will come with a price tag, one that causes us to lose what we worked for and hold dear.

But we need to remember that good things take time.

When we say yes to ourselves, our relationships change, the way we look at ourselves changes, and how we show up in every area of our lives shifts. I know time seems to pass so fast, and it feels like we've wasted so much, but that thinking is how we become impatient. And we lose a little faith. Or a lot.

Britt embodies the notion of ignoring the idea that you've wasted time. I have been with her on a few occasions when my younger self showed up to dispel an old story and give myself a chance to try something new. And in each situation, what she's offered me is truth with genuine love. No gimmicks, no advice, no "what I would do if I were you." Britt is a neuro psychotherapist and keynote speaker, so she's earned her stripes for having the right words. But her most significant gift, to me, is her humanness and outright honesty, which is some of the bravest I've ever witnessed.

While talking with Britt, I asked:

What did Little You always know was true?

Britt: That there was something bigger. Always. Something bigger than me. Something bigger than them [everyone]. Something bigger than what we could see. And I always felt very much a part of that bigness. Even when I was a kid. And it wasn't tied to religion. It was just tied to source.

> ### Get Curious
>
> What have you been part of in your life that was only as big and beautiful as it was because you said yes to you? How can you bring that bold, unique energy into your being today?

When you feel like you're locked in a cage you created for yourself, you might start politely asking for what you need, but after a while, you get in touch with the part of you that's tired, ready for change, and doesn't give a damn about politeness. You want what you want now. You've waited long enough. The claustrophobic feeling of being trapped begins to push you to demand something different. You start to move in a way you weren't willing to before and dream in a way you never thought you would again.

Maybe this is why people assume it's a crisis. Because there's such a desperation to it. You know you need a change, and you know you need it **now**.

While reading a study shared in *Frontiers in Psychology* on what helps us feel fulfilled in life, this quote struck me, "A fulfilled life is not a self-centered life."[1]

I know that many of us come from a lineage of generational growth stunting, where we've been asked, just like the ancestors who came before us, to please fall in line. Button up. And if you want something new that doesn't fit the generational cycle, please discard it before you step up to the plate. Somehow, someone who came before us got the idea that it was safest to do precisely what everyone before them had done. They put in place a set of rules that stopped the flow of new ideas or thoughts because that's all too tricky, too risky, and based on fantasy. But the idea that doing the least gets you the most is also a fantasy. When you choose not to live fully, you've decided those limiting rules are true. Be the person who finally stops the generational cycle, steps out of the line, and disrupts everything for your own good and all that comes after you.

You know your truth, the same truths that Little You held about you. And the bravest thing you'll do in your life is choose to move like you know what you know.

If you are halfway through your life, it's time to say yes to something other than a life half-lived. No matter where you are in your life, if what you've said yes to isn't working, it's time to be reacquainted with your self-trust and make the shift. It doesn't have to mean a new job. It doesn't have to mean divorce. Before you let your fears take over, let's think about how good this could be. Give yourself permission to go as big with your dreams as you do with your worries. Let's start small.

While talking with Britt, I shared:

So, at this point in your life, you're a therapist with more than ten thousand practicing hours, and you have a remembering that part of you has been waiting to step into the experience of performing in the circus. How does she come into alignment? How do you say yes?

Britt: Every summer when I was a kid growing up, my parents sent me to summer camp where I got to do circus stuff, and I loved it because it turned my brain off. There's nothing like flying upside down on scary things and spinning around in circles to silence the voices in your head.

And after many years of dealing with sexual trauma from childhood, sexual assault trauma in adulthood, domestic violence, drug addiction, after all of that, I think it was 2017 when I finally quit smoking cigarettes. That was the very last thing to go. And I was like, "Okay, well, now that I've cleared all of these chemicals, what do I want to do with myself?"

I went to a circus show in my city, and it was with students. It wasn't like this magical Cirque du Soleil. These were like Realtors, accountants, and lawyers—normal-looking humans. I had no idea this was even an option. So, I found a coach, signed up for lessons, and now, seven years later, I'm about to do a solo at a beautiful theater downtown, which is bananas.

P.S.: Britt did that solo and she absolutely killed it.

> **Get Curious**
>
> What have you told yourself isn't possible for you anymore because of age, timing, or some other belief that's kept you from saying yes? Do you still believe it's true? What is Little You still dreaming of?

The most beautiful thing about growing up is getting the chance to make the dreams of our little selves come true. Some of us have wept into our pillows, reciting prayers of hope. We've looked at ourselves in the mirror each morning, knowing there was more for us, determined to make it happen, but having no idea how. And some of us haven't realized that we're living our little selves' dreams every day because *we still don't feel complete.* The details of the dream may have changed, and the dream didn't come to be exactly as you envisioned, but if *you did it,* perhaps that's possible again.

I want you to remember that you are the Little You, right now, for the future, older you. This means you have an opportunity to bring seeds of hope to life for your future. I'm curious, what would your future look like if you could speak it right now? How will you slow down so you don't miss the blessings you've already created for yourself, that have gotten lost in the sameness of every day?

What did Little You know to be true? That curiosity was a gift. Little You knew that asking questions, feeling your rage, or letting yourself fall apart was a safe thing to do. For some of us, that truth was taken away, but you have the chance to get it back. Little You always knew that feeling disappointment or sadness wasn't a sign that all was ending. They knew it was a sign you were willing to burn it all down to build it back up. They knew whenever things became too much, you trusted yourself enough to feel hard feelings and release them before they found a home in you. Too many of us let pain reside within us, far outstaying its welcome.

If Little You could know what you wanted with clarity and deference, that means the you that exists today can too. What if you let it take the time it should take? What if you surrendered to the idea that you **do** know exactly what you're doing?

When making transformations, it's easiest to start as small as possible. Want to make it even easier? Do it with something you know you'll never skip. Listen to affirmations *while* brushing your teeth. Read or listen to one page from a book while you heat dinner. Remember, there's nothing wrong with feeling like change is **a lot**. Finding the easiest ways to get curious about what you want, and taking steps toward it, no matter how small, is a BIG win. The change you're seeking starts with saying yes in small ways. This is how you begin walking into your purpose.

Come Back to Yourself

Tonight, while getting your things ready for the next day, think about this: Imagine you're older, and reflecting on who you are today. What would no longer matter that feels like a big deal right now? Why do you think that is?

2 What If I Don't Have Enough Time?

You might be telling yourself that things seemed *easier* when you were younger, but I want you to get curious and ask yourself: Is that true? Yes, when you live through the lens of naivety, life does *feel* simpler. As we grow, we know it was false reassurance. Many of us suffered during our childhood and as young adults, but the innocence kept us feeling safe. It was a cloak of protection so we could grow. That safety is what allowed us to take risks, even with so many unknowns. That innocence is what made us feel like we had unlimited time, and that's a good thing. It made us willing to try *anything,* and gave us the willpower to figure out what we want.

Today, bravely stepping into the unknown feels riskier, because although we know we're not too late, we value our time and precious energy more. It wasn't easier to take risks back then; it was new.

Sometimes we romanticize the past without context. Truthfully, back then, we experienced the *both and*. It was both *exciting* and *challenging*. It was both *new* and *life changing*.

What if it's not "growing older" that's making you reassess what you commit yourself to, but instead the old rumblings of what you wanted calling out to you? What if you value yourself more today than you knew how to do then? Even though Little You had some clarity, they didn't have the authority. What if this life reassessment is YOU, today, coming to Little You's rescue?

A lot of us needed rescuing back then, and there was no one to do it.

— **Get Curious** —

How has Little You tried to save you?

Because of what I do for a living, when I ask people what's going on in their lives, I often get an honest answer. People stick a pin in the balloon of truth that's been floating above them, ready to burst, and let the words flow out unhinged. *I don't want to be married anymore. I don't like being a mom. I worry that I'll spend my life alone, even though I'm married. I hate that I have to take care of my parents when they never took care of me. I wish my daughter chose a real career, because I envisioned her moving out of the house sooner.* All the things people don't believe they can say to others are told to the healers, coaches, and therapists. No matter how many friends you have, no matter how close you are to your partner, there are some things you worry about saying out loud. Fear of burdening others, fear of being judged, and fear of being asked questions we're not ready to answer keep us quiet.

But when we share honestly, what lives in between those words we speak is a quest to reclaim our time. Had you known what you know now, would you have said yes? If you had more choice, freedom, flexibility, support, help . . . *if* there was *more*. Some of us are grateful we are looking forward, but some of us dream of going back. Back so we can be more honest with ourselves. Back to have the uncomfortable conversation that's created so much drama over the years. Back to choose our purpose and passions. We want one more chance to make the choice we couldn't make then, now that we have perspective. However, even when we're young adults, only twenty-five or twenty-six, with our whole lives ahead of us, we still feel the pull of time as we push to achieve goals.

But here's some reality regarding time.

According to data from the CDC, the average lifespan in the United States is approximately 80 years (technically 78.4 years),[1] and it's about the same, give or take a few years, based on the Office for National Statistics in the United Kingdom.

Using the CDC data, I decided to do some math of my own. This math doesn't account for how everyone sleeps, works, or lives, but using some hypothetical numbers, the following helped me understand how much time we might have for what we **want**, and I believe this encourages you to make a change in your life.

I calculated:

80-year lifespan: 700,800 hours
Sleep (7 hours a night): 204,400 hours

Work (55 hours per week for 54 years): 154,440 hours
That leaves you with 342,000 hours for everything
    else, which means . . .
You own 69 percent of your waking time

I know that some of us work fewer hours while others work way more. When I looked at research for work-life expectancy, the US Bureau of Labor Statistics[*] mentioned an average of 37.6 years in the workforce if you started at 16 years old. Still, it only accounts for years in the labor force, not calendar years from your first job to retirement. Plus, the study hasn't been updated since *1986,* and we both know that things have changed drastically economically since then. People are working harder and *longer.* I rounded the number of working years up to 54 years because I didn't want to limit labor to full-time work only. I tried to account for all the *labor* that many of us experience from a young age: caring for siblings, part-time jobs, summer jobs, and other responsibilities. These are symbolic numbers that are different for every individual, but follow me for a minute.

What does this show us?

Using these hypothetical numbers, it shows that throughout our lives, we own about 69 percent of our waking hours.

Now you could whittle this number down to account for your specific details, such as commuting time, additional work, and adulting, etc. But theoretically, even with numbers on the higher end, you may still own about 50 percent of awake time. These numbers were shocking to me.

---

[*] US Bureau of Labor Statistics. (1986, February). "Worklife estimates: Effects of race and education." Retrieved from https://www.bls.gov/opub/reports /worklife-estimates/archive/worklife-estimates-1986.pdf.

I'll admit when I—ever the optimist—calculated this, it excited me. I couldn't wait to share it with people, and I don't know why, but I expected to hear excitement because to me, this meant we had more time than we maybe thought. To me, this meant we needed to make different choices so our time was spent the way we wanted. Perhaps, if we committed to changing some things around, we'd get to experience the fruit of our boundaries and then some. But that isn't how anyone saw this data, and I don't know what I was thinking.

Friends and colleagues struck me down, sharing that they wanted to change, but they had too many errands, too many kids, and too many responsibilities. Too much going on to even find the time to watch a favorite show, let alone go on an adventure with their "waking hours." They told me to take that fluffy *55 hours of work time* somewhere else, because they were working two jobs or were nonstop with their kids at home. Even those without kids, partners, or excessive responsibilities expressed how the world felt so heavy that time seemed to be moving on a conveyor belt where someone had pressed *fast forward.* Everyone told me to take my data and shove it because it wouldn't and doesn't mean a thing.

I honestly understand their reactions because the world is going through *a lot,* and so are we. People are overwhelmed and struggling to function in the most basic ways. Being told *you have more time* feels like toxic positivity and is the opposite of what people want to hear. People want to be validated in their experience of struggling, not have more steps or reframes thrown their way. However, and I mean this, I'm not sharing this data to try to make it "all better." I'm sharing this so the next time you wonder why you haven't done what you wanted, you don't mundanely blame *time* and believe your life must stay the way that it is. I feel so strongly that my job is to ensure you know there might be other options to make your life better.

I also know that people don't want to hear that they have more time than they think because then they have to face the uncomfortable question: If I have more time, why am I not spending it the way I want? I know we can't control everything and I know change is hard. But be honest with yourself. When you *do* have the time, are you spending it the way you want to? And if not, who, if not you, can change that?

Amanda grew up dreaming of having it better than her little version, and she began working at a young age, doing all she could to succeed *fast*. It's one of the things I admire the most about her story, because like many of us, she pushed herself knowing hard work was part of the game, but she never pretends any of it came easily. She mentioned, *"I prided myself on being a machine, and that's what I was rewarded for."*

I know a lot of recovering perfectionists, people pleasers, oldest daughters/children, parentified kids, and overachievers who relate to this. The better, shinier, and more exceptional you are, the more you're seen and hopefully loved. But whether it gets you closer to your goal or not, you're working yourself into the ground. You think you're trying to win, but present you is trying to save younger you. All you wanted was to be free, so you fight and push, just like Amanda did, like I did, and like so many of us, hoping this was the way to rescue ourselves. However, the long hours caught up to Amanda quickly and unexpectedly.

While talking with Amanda, I shared:

You mentioned burnout, and I know for everyone, there's a moment where you're just working too much. But for you, it seemed to be a combination of three things: working too much, not being aligned with your soul's purpose, and doing too much partying, etc.

What was the moment when you felt like you had to get out, when you knew something had to change? When did you know?

Amanda: When I experienced my extreme burnout, I wasn't listening to my body every day. My body listened to me every day. I said to myself, "You're going to get up. You're going to work twenty hours today. If you have to be on the floor in high heels until four in the morning, so be it. We'll take a Tylenol PM in the cab on the way home and two shots of espresso in the morning, three more when you get to the office." So, for me, I didn't burn out. My heart stopped functioning.

Amanda's story teaches us many things. First, it highlights how we sometimes build habits when we're young that weren't helpful **but worked**. And because they worked then, we keep doing them now, even if they harm us, because we don't know another way. Secondly, it highlights the way we might judge ourselves or others for the way we learned to survive, even though we were doing the best we could.

You might be reading this thinking it's an extreme and unrelatable story. Maybe you're saying you would never be out until four in the morning, using coffee and Tylenol PM to help you rise and rest. Maybe you're wondering how this relates to your purpose. But remember, so many of us grew up outside of conventional ideals, carrying a story of resilience, not by choice, but because we had to.

Single parents, caretakers, people working multiple jobs, people who served in the military, and people trying to create a life for themselves through their work often have stories that feel extreme to others. We were committed to doing anything to change our story, not knowing that this pace of work would disconnect us from ourselves and our purpose. The reality is most of us have lived a situation where we ignored the messages our bodies were giving us in the name of saving ourselves. It's incredibly brave to decide to be your own hero.

Amanda continues:

I went to the gynecologist to refill my birth control, and she goes, "You need to go to the cardiologist right now." And I was like, "What are you talking about?" She's like, "Amanda, your pulse is completely erratic. You need to go." I'm twenty-eight years old and I'm like, "What are you talking about?" And this woman's literally saying, "I will not write you a prescription for birth control until you go to the cardiologist." And I was like, "M*****f*****, I've got to get back to the office."

I didn't want to hear it. I literally said, "What? You're crazy." But I went to the cardiologist because I needed my birth control. And they had me wear a heart monitor, which you wear for seven days. And after that, they were like, "Amanda, your heart arrhythmia is so severe that you need to get heart surgery. Your heart is skipping every third beat." And I was pissed. I was ashamed. I was annoyed. I was like, I don't need this. In my mind, at that age, I was thinking, *I need to get 30 Under 30.* That was my mindset. I'm twenty-eight. I can't put the pause button on now.

And I literally delayed the surgery because I was getting married in March and then we were opening a venue at work in May. I told my doctor I can get it the weekend after we open the venue. I waited almost six months.

Me: Oh my God.

Amanda: If you had known me back then, this is how crazy I was. I was like, I cannot get heart surgery until after we open this nightclub because I need to make sure this happens. I literally scheduled it for Memorial Day weekend. As the date approached, the reality sunk in more and more that I can't keep going like this. I had no one around me telling me, "Slow down." It actually makes me sad thinking about it now. I had no one around me saying, "Oh my God, this is happening to you." No one was worried about me. No one was saying, "There's another way." I had no good advice. No angels on my shoulder. My fiancé and I were so in the struggle, so in survival mode, and neither of us had the maturity or financial wherewithal to say, "Amanda, slow down." We didn't have the maturity to understand what I was going through, what we were going through. And honestly, even if he had said to slow down, I wouldn't have listened because it was me against the world. We needed my job.

How many of you have put off a doctor's appointment to prioritize what felt more critical? People have hidden pregnancies from employers, fearful of losing their position.

People have waited for essential procedures because they lacked insurance to cover them and had to work instead. Or people have chosen others over their health.

The anger that comes up around this reality stems from society ignoring our needs. People aren't a priority. And when there's no one on your side, it's harder to choose yourself. You may not even know what it is to choose yourself.

Amanda continued:

And then, I remember my bosses being like, "We're all on heart medication."

Me: No!

Amanda: Oh, yeah. When I went in to say that I was taking a sabbatical, they were like, "Are you sure? I'll give you the number to my cardiologist, they're on the Upper East Side." And I was like, "No, I don't think I'm going that route." So, I took a sabbatical. We moved down to New Orleans. I went to India. I did the whole f****** thing before *Eat, Pray, Love* was out. I went to Bali. I did all the things, you know?

What's funny is if you said to me when I was twenty-five or twenty-six years old "I have a magic wand, what would you want to do in life?" It's very much what I'm doing now.

But if you asked me "Well, why don't you do it?" I would have laughed in your f****** face. I had no faith in myself. I had no thought that creating this type of reality was possible. I thought, *okay, maybe one day*, but it felt like there was no chance it was possible because I was already sowing the seeds of working in healing and spirituality, my dream, but it was always only a hobby, you know?

> ## Get Curious
>
> Have there been times when you've pushed yourself beyond what was comfortable to reach your goals? In hindsight, what did you learn? Was it ever worth it? Would you do it again? And ultimately, what was the price (spiritually, emotionally, etc.)?

CAN I SHARE A HARD TRUTH?

If you identified with the friends and colleagues who struck down my math, I'm not mad at you. I relate. But I was hoping you could do me (and you) a favor. Put aside everything you spend time on that's entirely out of your control: taxes, caretaker responsibilities for parents, health issues, etc. There are many things thrust upon us that we can't say no to or choose not to do. That's not your fault, and still, the burden is yours.

Okay, hard truth time. Please look at the things in your life you have taken on that don't belong to you. The over-giving, the codependent relationships, the lack of boundaries, and the choices that were (and maybe still are) entirely yours to say no to, but instead you said yes. For many of us, we had no idea that the yes would take up so much time. I agree and hear you, but it was still your yes. These yeses are keeping you from dedicating time to your art, your passions, your joy. This self-inquiry truly matters.

Accepting the part you play in deciding where your time goes is an integral part of this process, because it also means you'll recognize the power of stopping things in their tracks by saying no the first time in the future. You can love pets, but know you don't have the time for another one. You can dream of having a bigger family, but understand you don't have the capacity to raise more children. No is hard, but necessary to keep you aligned. Life happens, of course, and we can't control everything. But when you *can* be in the driver's seat, and you find yourself having the opportunity to choose? Please be honest and choose as if you're the person left with the consequences.

After conducting this research, I continued to dig, because as much as we need to choose wisely now and in the future, we also have to acknowledge that some of us are too burned out to make any choice, let alone "the right choice." In my opinion, burnout is a close companion of time.

Amanda's story is more common than we think, and although burnout manifests in the body differently for everyone, when it manifests physically, it usually does so loudly.

Frenetic burnout, which is most likely the type Amanda experienced and the version we're often taught about, isn't the only kind of burnout. In research published by *BMC Public Health*,[2] they found burnout can be classified into three clinical subtypes:

Frenetic Burnout: Experienced by people who are highly ambitious and take on excessive workloads

If you spend much of your time working to "make it," you might make a lot of money, have a successful business, and check all the boxes. I'm not saying don't go after your dreams, but I want you to get curious about what else you might be saying yes to when you overdo it. Long working hours mean you won't have much time for the part of your life that includes friends, rest, and your interests. Overworking some-times means you're hoping to find validation in what you're doing versus in who you are. I also know sometimes you're doing what you need to do so you can pay bills, but this type of burnout shows up for those who overwork to achieve. It's important to note sometimes we have the insatiable desire to succeed and thrive because at one point in your life you were barely surviving. Our past can lead us to form new habits with the hope of breaking old cycles, but we don't realize that what we've said yes to is a new, harsh pattern. Don't judge the ways you tried to free yourself; get curious.

Taking on more than you can handle usually signals a problem with boundaries. If you do this in excess, and it leads to burnout, even if you're checking all those boxes you planned, you probably won't feel like you're leading a meaningful life. You'll be tired, overwhelmed, overworked, and most likely feel alone. You'll wonder why giving yourself everything you wanted isn't turning into the feeling of fulfill-ment you envisioned. It's not that hard work isn't essential, but working isn't all there is.

Underchallenged Burnout: Experienced by people who aren't challenged enough in their roles and often feel dissatisfied, lack professional growth, and may even become bored

How many times have you been at a job where you were micromanaged, belittled, not given clear direction, not al-lowed to grow in your role, and left every day feeling dread at going back the next? Yes, some people don't care to work, but when I say this next thing I'm about to say, I'm not talking about them. When you see an office filled with people who aren't focused, who don't take tasks seriously, and who don't even care who knows it, I always think about under-challenged burnout.

When you don't feel validated, seen, and appreciated at work, it influences how you feel about yourself too. And when you're not being challenged professionally, that feeling of genuine boredom can leak out into every area of your life. Yes, we want things to feel easier, but we like accomplishing things that feel impossible. We like overcoming. We like being trusted to follow through. We need work environments where we're seen as people who can be respected and trusted to do our jobs.

Worn-out Burnout: Experienced by people who've given up because the stress and lack of control have made them feel helpless

Think toxic work environments, people who are worn out from working more than one job, and jobs that require excessive work to survive. Some jobs are fortified by drama, demanding bosses, unprofessionalism, and fear-based management that create an environment filled with stress. There are many things beyond our control in our jobs, but every day should not feel like a shot in the dark.

When you look at time through the eyes of a person experiencing burnout, yes, many of us own the majority of our waking hours, but if the time we spend at work is so miserable that all we can think about is crawling right into bed: *It doesn't matter that we own our waking hours if our job is taking the light and life out of us.* We won't feel empowered to do anything in our downtime if we're trying to fill ourselves back up enough to get back to work. The same is true for emotionally draining relationships.

Where we spend our time impacts how we feel in every area of our lives.

A research study published in *Frontiers in Psychology* titled "Spillover and Crossover of Exhaustion and Life Satisfaction Among Dual-Earner Parents,"[3] demonstrated that your feelings about work can spill over into all other areas of your life. In short, if you feel great at work, your relationships could reflect that satisfaction. On the other hand, if you're stressed, your relationships could reflect that too.

I know many systems in modern society make it difficult to have your own time, and the dismantling of them would certainly change things. If we had villages supporting moms, if you only worked one job and were paid a living wage, if healthcare were easier, and so on. Let's keep these realities that need to be shifted in mind, but also do what we can with what we have right now.

> ### Get Curious
>
> When you think about the time you're not working, not doing, not adulting—how much do you spend the way you want? How much of your time do you believe you own? Does it feel like any of these burnouts need to be explored with a therapist, coach, or healer?

I know an internal story might exist that says my kids, my partner, my life don't allow me to have time for myself.

I believe you, I know it's hard . . . and I still want you to get curious. Where is it true and where is it not?

Where have you chosen your comforts, even if they aren't what you want, over curiosity? Because our comforts aren't always cozy. Our comforts are what we're used to. And in a world of chaos and lack of control, sometimes what we're used to feels safer than any new unknown.

Those numbers about our time don't mean you or I are bad stewards of our time and that we're the problem. I'm also not diagnosing you with burnout; I don't have the qualifications to do so. What I know is we have at least three generations of exhausted people: Gen X, Millennials, and even Gen Z. We're craving *ease*. We've survived unprecedented event after unprecedented event, and yes, we're resilient, but resilience comes at a cost.

If we're not consciously choosing how we use our time, then our lives may be passing us by. I hope that understanding is highlighted. If we got curious enough, and slowed down enough, to give ourselves a deeper level of awareness of what we're doing, perhaps we'd choose something different. Maybe we'd see a solution where we always saw a wall. Possibly, one small change could help us feel less stuck, and our lives would feel more meaningful. But if we don't get curious, we may never know.

And listen, bring your skeptical self to the discussion. Love on that part of you too. We both know that skeptical part's been keeping you safe with their questions and side-eyeing. Just promise you won't allow doubt to keep you from what's possible. Promise yourself right now that you'll give yourself a chance, okay?

I love how Amanda shares her experience of giving herself a chance to do something new:

Amanda: I started teaching yoga, and everything was beautiful, right?

No.

I went from making six figures a year to making four figures. I was broke, but I was back in New York and I needed an employer for my rental application.

I set boundaries at my job, and I realized, wow, they still like and respect me. Once stable, I started looking for jobs in the wellness industry because I'm a good businesswoman, and I wanted to find a job where I was still a businesswoman doing marketing, business development, and strategy, but instead of in nightlife, in wellness.

So that year changed me; it wasn't the final step, but it changed me.

Remember, boundaries are the rules you put in place telling people how they can (or can't) treat you. They aren't negotiations or ultimatums. They're a mechanism for respect and love in your relationships. Those small boundaries Amanda set led to the life she lives today, helping women in business, primarily founders who are overworked and overwhelmed, get the support they need for their businesses with her experience in marketing and strategy, while also calming their nervous systems. She is working in her absolute genius zone, and escaped the city for country life. Back then, Amanda would've never thought what she has today was possible. But even when she had no clue what would come next, she bet on herself, and it's so beautiful to see her enjoy the fruits of all that labor.

> ### Get Curious
>
> What story do you tell yourself about boundaries that keeps you from choosing what you need? Are you okay with your next step not being your final step?

Writing your bucket list requires time. Looking for new jobs involves time. Going for a walk involves time. And we don't receive instant proof that it was worth it. Amanda didn't—it took time. In addition to needing time to do the things we want, it *takes time* to learn it was worth the commitment, and that's a risk too.

It's hard to give our all to anything that doesn't feel guaranteed. I get it. But if you've read this and any of this has started to set your thoughts in motion about another way . . . follow it. It won't be clear at first, but follow it. It won't make sense at first, but follow it.

This is where you build your trust. This is where you reconnect with your knowing.

This is where the work to come back to yourself is done.

> ### Come Back to Yourself
>
> For one week, while brushing your teeth in the evening, think about how you spent your time that day. Ask yourself: If I had the power to change one thing about today, what would I shift? If I had the power to do one thing all day today, what would it be?

this is the era,
where you learn your worth
your silent dreams
begin to speak.
this is your era,
where you make your move.
your dreams are waiting on you.
your life is waiting on you.
bet on you.

3 What Am I Pretending I Don't Know?

I know you've met people who seem to know exactly what they're here to do.

I also know this seems like the goal: to understand what you're *here* for. You want to look at yourself and, without a shadow of a doubt, feel how *you were born for this very moment.* You want to feel the tingly feeling we experience when we see someone living their gifts out loud. Everyone does.

We all have multiple gifts. But we don't always give ourselves the chance to try them. When we choose something safe and define ourselves and our lives by those choices, our gifts that never got to shine don't go away. And after living awhile, you remember that those gifts are a huge part of who you are. Still, you may say to those very precious gifts, the ones you think about but haven't used, that you'll get to them *one day*. Eventually, your gifts stop believing you'll come back. And you stop believing you'll come back for them, and the ache gets stronger.

Purpose relies on courage to survive. Without courage, we'd never be willing to create what we haven't seen. It should leave you in awe, when you think about how much courage it's taken to commit to things you didn't know were possible. First person to graduate from college. First person to start a business. Courage helps you bypass fear, giving you the strength to *confront* the voices within and around you that try to stop you. It also ignores the part of you that wants to quit because it feels too hard. Even if you aren't the first in your community to do something, getting started still takes a ton of courage, because you already saw firsthand that it's going to take a lot of guts, time, and dedication. After you give it your all, it may not work out, and despite knowing this, you still go for it. That's courage.

I also want to name that *purpose is **not** a destination*. We won't "arrive" at what we're here to do and be stuck there forever. People will come and go, circumstances will change, we'll be asked to grow when we're not ready, and we'll be asked to stay when all we want to do is run away. Purpose is an invitation to lifelong transformation that asks you to be willing to leave it all for something new, something greater, something that needs the very thing that you have and were made to do. Your purpose will ask too much of you sometimes, and at the worst moments. Your purpose will stretch you, when all you want to do is rest. Again, purpose is *always* an invitation. You get to decide, and yet, it won't make it easy to say no.

Whether you're the person with the blueprint in hand or

you're the person doing it all for the first time, we tend to question ourselves. *Do I have what it takes? What if it doesn't work out? Who do I think I am?*

I know many people don't face imposter syndrome, and I think that's great; more power to you if this isn't part of your human experience. But a lot of us do. However, I don't believe imposter syndrome fully encompasses the experience we're having when we don't bring all of us to the table. I believe we morph into the version of our little selves that couldn't shine too brightly, the version that had to hide. Pretending is one of the tools that Little You knew best. Yes, kids are imaginative when it's time to dream big, and they also pretend when it feels like the safest way to hide.

> ### Get Curious
>
> What are you pretending you don't know to be true about who you are, so other people stay comfortable?

Growing up in New York City, I rode the train daily, and it's always been a place where I could sort out what's on my mind.

But when you ride the train, you pay attention because there are signs everywhere. Signs telling you whether the train is going downtown or uptown, express or local. In addition to signs, there are usually announcements. There are large, lit-up boards that share the status of every train for hours. Once you step on the train, you'll hear additional announcements from the conductor, so if you don't pay attention, you might find yourself yanking off your headphones to hear why you see people running off the train. Did it just become express? Is there a rat? What's going on?

Commuting on the train is a complex system, like life. There are so many ways to get to the same place. There are so many opportunities to get lost and a lot of distractions.

Sometimes, we get on our metaphorical trains intending to ride the path toward creating a peaceful family. When things start going wrong, instead of shifting, we start pretending and ignoring reality. Instead of making decisions knowing we deserve better, we keep riding. When we keep riding, the announcements start blaring over our internal PA system. At first, we hear encouraging words, telling us we deserve better and that we should make a change. But the longer we ignore the truth, the more those announcements shift from encouraging to damaging, because we stop believing we deserve it. We start hearing repeated conversations from parents and friends, saying *I told you so*. We ride along, hearing their worries, their fears, and gripes. Our disappointments grow louder the longer we stay seated on the train that is now going in the wrong direction. With all the chatter, we grow overwhelmed, and it's easy to get lost in the noise.

When you stop believing in yourself, you stop riding to the destination you wanted. You somehow transfer to the *I'm going to pretend I don't know who I am* train. Or perhaps lack of self-belief causes you to get on the *I'm okay with staying small* train. Or maybe you get lost for years, and board the *Who do you think you are* train. The train is moving what feels like *forward,* but you're no longer headed where you intended to go. It keeps you in a delusional trance, believing that movement is progress, but if it's not aligned movement, then you're moving further away from your truth. You're moving further away from the real you.

It's easier to pretend and perform through life because that ensures we'll fit in. We are conditioned to live life the way others want us to. When we meet someone whose family supports their artistic dreams, or when we come across someone who stands confidently in their choice not to have kids, get married, or do anything conventional because they don't want to, we gasp. *How did you know that you were allowed to choose? How did you know that you could do something different than what everyone else is doing?*

It's one of two things. They were brought up in an environment that supported them, and they never had to forget who they were to be accepted. Or they decided to stop pretending and choose for themselves anyway.

Once you stop pretending, you realize you're bigger than you ever imagined. You know your heart can hold more love, that disappointment won't stop you, that people may not like you when you choose to be whole, and that you might lose them. If you lose them, you learn you'll be okay. Yes, you may have to start again. But when you stop pretending, you discover that getting another chance isn't a curse, it's a gift.

Use this gift.

Stop pretending not to know what lights you up.

Stop pretending not to know what you want to do more of.

Stop pretending not to know what you'd be doing right now if you could.

Remember, you've only pretended not to know because it's so hard to admit that you always knew and *still* didn't choose you.

But we've all ignored our truth at one time or another.

And you probably ignored it because it didn't align with what you'd been told to do.

Or you ignored your truth . . .

because you wanted to fit in.

because you're afraid "it" wouldn't work.

because you got distracted.

because taking up space is too scary.

because you're tired.

because you have no idea where to begin.

Or you're waiting for the right time to say the uncomfortable thing, and then something happened, and you felt trapped, and years went by. But no matter the reason, remember that **you know**.

I know there were times in your life when you went along with what you knew you shouldn't, and when everything hit the fan, you said, *I knew this would happen*, and the truth is, you did.

You knew this wasn't the career for you.

You knew that wasn't the marriage or relationship for you.

You knew *they* weren't ever really your friend.

You knew "it" wasn't supposed to feel this way.

But like we all do at one time or another, we ignore our gut.

So, how can we choose to act on what we know and stop pretending?

While talking with Britt, I asked:

Me: I'm wondering, what did Little You always know to be true?

Britt: That adults aren't really a thing. It's not defined by age. It's a state of being. I don't live in my adult self all the time. You've seen me slide into different younger parts.

But I think my little self knew adulthood is a total myth. You can go your whole life and never get to adulthood.

Me: Wow, so in your opinion, what happens if you don't get to adulthood?

Britt: I think adolescence is supposed to be the bridge that transitions you from childhood to adulthood. And if you don't have skillful parents and resources, you get stuck on that bridge and you never fully cross over. I'm forty-four and I feel like I'm just now getting a glimpse of the land of adulthood, and it's awesome. This whole "I don't want to be an adult" thing I do not subscribe to. Being an adult is awesome. Being a kid is terrible. You have no power. You have no agency. You're dependent upon everyone and everything.

I also think what we call adulthood is often a bunch of adolescents masquerading as grown-up people. The secret key that unlocks the transition to adulthood is grief. And as a culture we suck at grief. Even if you had an awesome childhood, you don't get to be a kid anymore. So, you have to grieve that. And if you had a crappy childhood, you don't get to go redo it. So, you have to grieve that. But grief is the key that unlocks the world of adulthood. That sounds morbid, but it's actually really empowering.

When we think about grief, we don't often think about disappointment, but pretending disappointment doesn't exist can be a barrier to starting again. Admitting those hard feelings helps us learn how to make different choices. Being hard on ourselves keeps us stuck. Fear of disappointment becomes a barrier to truth and transformation. Allowing ourselves to feel disappointment is what invites us to grieve.

Something we wanted so badly that we were willing to pretend, hide, and lose ourselves to gain isn't going to happen. When we're disappointed—in life, in ourselves, in the world, in our families, in the way things turned out, in the time we lost—sometimes we stop trusting our knowing. We think, *if I've always known, then how could I choose this?* We stop trusting our little selves. We stop looking at our dreams, promises, and hopes. It all hurts too much. But pretending we never knew? That feels like a balm because **if we never knew, then we never betrayed ourselves.** It's a painful distraction, but it's time to remember.

I've shared this before, but wisdom unfortunately doesn't come with age. You have to *want* to learn and accept the lessons. When you find yourself riding on the *Who do you think you are train*, you must be willing to show up ready to remind that internal voice that you are exactly who you think you are.

Someone who has big dreams of who you're going to be in the world.

Someone who wants more and is willing to ask for it.

Someone who found out life can chew you up and spit you out, but it's not the end.

Someone who doesn't know if you have what it takes to keep showing up, but you're gonna keep going.

To get out of your stuckness, be willing to feel the grief, the disappointment, and the feelings that are yours. This is humanness. You only learn resilience by allowing yourself to lean in to the challenging moments. I know we're tired of building resilience; that's a disappointing reality of adult life too. We don't share how much it takes to get up every morning while going through your own stuff, let alone everyone else in your life's stuff; and we haven't even added on the world's stuff. Humanness is crying, sharing, working through challenging moments, and then choosing to get back up.

For most of us, we forget that we don't have to ride the train alone. We pretend we don't know that we don't have to do life solo, but that's also to try to protect ourselves from being let down. With community, grief, disappointment, failure, and humanness aren't so burdensome. We share each other's experiences, and we get to love on each other; for many of us, in ways we've never experienced before. For many, you're healing your younger self by choosing to be fully present as your bigger self today.

Get Curious

What are you pretending you don't know? To be clear, I don't want you to uproot your life, unless you want to. There's no pressure to find anything if you feel like you know it all right now. But if you know your truth, what's keeping you from taking a step?

I'd love for you to write a letter from yourself today to Little You, with the wisdom and hindsight you have right now. What love notes would you share? This might be the thing you need to read to remind yourself that you are beautiful, bright, deserving, and a light. All of that is still true about you.

Let the words from this letter play over the internal PA system on that train you've been riding, to give you the strength to take the smallest step toward choosing a new train, a new path. All leading back to what you've always wanted, to your purpose.

On the other side of this small next step lies the next challenge. But that *one day* that you've been waiting for, to finally meet your gifts and give yourself what you want, is on the other side of that next small step.

By saying yes to your gifts, you put yourself in the power position to reclaim what has always been yours.

> ### Come Back to Yourself
>
> Find a picture of yourself at the age you envisioned your little self a few chapters back. Put the image in a place you will see every day; maybe on your bathroom mirror, or as your phone wallpaper. Ask yourself these questions as you continue to read: What did Little You have back then that you need now? What did that version of you need that you can give yourself today by choosing a new path? Spend time with whichever question feels more important to you, and remember, you get to choose.

this is the era
that you bask in all your blessings,
knowing the roots you come from
have always been rich.
you come from good earth,
the kind that runs deep.
from you, all things grow.
Good. Things. Take. Time.

4 What If I'm the Reason I'm Unhappy?

By now, I hope the stories you've been carrying about your life are unraveling under the magnifying glass of curiosity. The closer you look, the clearer it becomes.

Remember, *your clarity might not come with answers*. It's okay not to have solutions for your stories and just be present to them.

For some of us, the stories we've carried are deeply rooted, grounded into our bodies like a two-hundred-year-old oak tree, and depending on the story, it could, generationally, be that old. We might be carrying a belief that *this is how it is for everyone in my family*, and that memory-like belief can feel immovable. The story was passed down to live through us, even though we never experienced it ourselves.

Since we don't always choose the stories we carry, their

presence is explained with new stories—ones like, our parents failed us. Our teachers failed us. Mentors, first employers, professors. They all failed us. They gave us plans to follow without enough instructions. Their rules were put in place without discussion. They provided a sense of structure while we grew but never shared the why. We were expected to follow our caretakers mindlessly, believing they were keeping something from us, a truth we were too young to understand. But the real reason they never shared *the why* is because they didn't know what they were doing either. We had expectations for the adults in our lives that could never be fulfilled because *they were still growing.* When things don't work out, we point our fingers, trying to figure out why we didn't get the truth.

> ── **Get Curious** ──
>
> If your mentors, caretakers, or parents had shared their truth, "I don't know what I'm fully doing either," could the story you carry about the truth be broken? If they shared *what they knew to be true*, in hindsight, would it have made life easier for you?

When working with people in groups or one-on-one settings, most share that they wish they would have received the *pull-back-the-curtain truth* while growing up. However, I think we hope receiving the truth back then would help us avoid the pain and heartache we're experiencing now. The truth doesn't always save us from harsh reality.

You can't go back, but you can admit that you needed to be able to say to your caretakers:

Tell me you will walk this path with me, and I won't be alone in my fears and uncertainty.

Tell me you'll be on my side as I learn hard lessons.

Tell me if I don't choose to do what you want for me, that I'll still have your love and acceptance.

I believe having space to say these words could've freed a lot of us. And maybe it still can.

Instead of hearing those responses, many of us were surrounded by adults with unprocessed traumas and internalized limitations, which they projected onto us. It didn't feel safe to speak the truth, even if our childhoods were wonderful. These old stories were so alive, they were like an additional family member, always present at every event, in all the pictures, loudly beaming through us, a string of stories we never spoke of but that were often spoken through us.

We're asked to make do and *be happy* with what we got from our childhood, even when it wasn't enough. So, when I ask, *are you the reason you're unhappy?*, I'm sure the first natural response is *absolutely not*. Or more likely, *hell no. How could I be? Look at my circumstances. Look at what I was given. Look at what I had to survive to be where I am today.*

I see you and I know life can sometimes feel like a fight. Swing after swing, round after round, you're expected to get up and go back out there. You're expected to perform, get beaten up, and win in the end. I know sometimes you don't feel like you have what it takes. I know you wish it could be easier. And I know you're doing what you can.

When feelings of how hard life is surface, this is when it seems easier to *pretend you don't know who you are*. And this is how you end up living a miserable life. Even if you didn't get what you needed, there's still time to give it to yourself now.

I know too well that we forget how lessons often lead to opportunities. We forget that those moments of fighting in life are training us for greater things. Every fight isn't intended to tear you apart. Some fights equip you with the skills you need to win. But without people around us ensuring that we're supported through these moments, we feel attacked. When we learn to lean on those two-hundred-year-old oak tree–like stories we carry, we can remember we're not just carrying memories of grief and stories of pain, but memories of nourishment, strength, and love. Your roots have always been rich. If no one around you had the language to tell you this then, remember that truth now.

You can't go back and be the little person you were, encouraging the adults who raised you to give you the truth about what you carry, and honestly, you probably wouldn't have listened anyway. My grandmother always showered me with lessons I keep close, but back then, I didn't value how expensive those gifts were. It's only in hindsight that I see they are gold.

The human spirit craves lessons. If you're honest while being curious, you'll see how you're often in your way, blocking your happiness. This isn't what you're supposed to say, and honestly, I wouldn't have said this a few years ago myself. I would've found any reason, excuse, or explanation possible to help you hold a light on the wrongs you experienced and blame *someone else*. I would've shouted from the mountaintops as I stood next to you, "Life would be different if everyone did what they were supposed to do."

Because truthfully, the harmful behaviors we've learned aren't just *our fault*, and it sucks that we're the ones forced to do the cleanup. Trust me, I know, but this is our **big** life now.

If you're ready to stop listening to the same stories making you feel down and depleted, you must take accountability for the years, choices, and situations that belong to you. There are so many moments ahead, waiting for you to choose something different. It isn't too late. You're not too late.

Please conserve your energy, because life is like a boxing match. It takes energy to hold both hands up while you're waiting for the next punch to come your way. It takes energy to gather yourself as you prepare for the next round, which may be just as intense as the last. You'll need mental strength to decide that, despite the fight you're in, you *still* want to walk out of the ring soft and willing, not hardened by the things that tried to break you. To be human in that ring, empathy and compassion must be with you.

To bring empathy with you in the ring, forget about winning every match. Life is asking, *can you practice?* Can you show up uncertain but ready? This is how you get out of your way. This is how hard lessons become breakthroughs. Even if you lose your footing, lose this round, lose this match, you know there's still next time. It feels like it's the match of your life, but if you're still standing at the end, it was just another practice round.

The other option is to go over every missed hit. Blame the referee. Focus on the skills you never received. Put your energy into what life would've been like if you were afforded what your friends *appeared* to have. Tell yourself that you missed out. Put all your energy into the negative only.

To be very clear, yes, you deserve accountability; it's essential. You deserved everything and more in the past, and you still do. You deserve the apologies you may never receive. And you never deserved any harm, abuse, or shame.

"**And.**" This is the brilliant word you'll be adding to your vocabulary if it doesn't already exist. They didn't prepare you, AND you can decide to find ways to prepare yourself. They didn't know what to do, AND now you've decided you're ready to learn. They didn't prioritize you, AND you decided you were ready to break that generational cycle.

It didn't start the way it should've for Little You, AND you have the power to change that now.

So, let's go back to the question at hand. Are you the reason you're unhappy?

You know your story. It's not easy to admit that you've been in your way, and every part of you might be calling me all sorts of names right now. But if you're in your way, it's not on purpose. I know that doesn't make it feel any less crappy.

I'm not asking you to blame yourself, I'm asking you to practice healthy accountability. Accountability stops us from making the same choices repeatedly and is the very practice that allows our lessons to become blessings. For example, if you look at your dating history and say, "I always choose the wrong people, I don't know what's wrong with me. I never make good choices," that's self-blame. That statement isn't helping you learn your patterns, it's just pointing out what you believe you did wrong. If instead you said, "I can see how I've consistently chosen people who aren't right for me, and it's because I was always hoping I could fix what I knew was wrong. Now I know I'm not their *fixer,* I'm their *partner.* I deserve better and will choose like I do next time." In that scenario, you're still being honest about your part in the pattern, but you're approaching it with care, not with harm. This makes all the difference.

You might be thinking: Why would I do, say, and be things to myself that aren't helpful?

I'm not making excuses when I say this because the truth is, you didn't know any different. You used the tools available and did the best you could to make it all work. You tried pretending, you tried forgetting, you tried burning out, you tried it all. You've been working so hard to give yourself the life you deserve. Instead of tearing yourself apart, show yourself gratitude because you've tried to protect yourself and keep it together the best way you knew how. Now, you can give yourself the gift of living your life like you know what truly matters to you, and why not start with joy?

While I was talking with Lia, she shared:

Lia: I find it interesting that a lot of people I know, for the first half of their life are really contemplating purpose and meaning, and then the second half of their life, they're like f*** purpose. What about joy? What about pleasure, right? I don't think I was integrating joy and pleasure into my purpose until I started to reach midlife, but now, I'm starting to think about what if fun was part of my purpose? What if I asked myself what would bring me laughter?

Get Curious

What does "joy" mean to you? I know it can be hard to find joy when so much is happening around us. But what would it feel like to get out of the fight and into the joy of life energy?

There used to be a time when fun was a priority in your life. You probably didn't feel happy all day, every day, but you had fun whenever you could.

Your life was lit up when you thought about the people you might spend time with, the things you might get to see, and the places you might get to go. Remember? You spent more time dreaming up what inspired you than naming all the reasons your dreams could never come true. And your dreams were not only tied to your career. They were about you too.

I'm talking about play. Race-your-friend-in-the-streets, watch-a-movie-and-laugh-out-loud, try-a-new-recipe, get-together-unexpectedly, browse-a-bookstore, go-window-shopping, play-a-card-game kind of play.

If you're missing play, you're missing purpose. It's time to get out of your way.

> ### Get Curious
>
> When was the last time you were bent over laughing? If you can't remember the last time you felt giddy, consider whether you've sub-scribed to a version of adulthood that doesn't include enjoyment.

I researched to understand more about how play might impact us, and I learned that when we play, we activate the Default Mode Network (DMN) in the brain.[1] The DMN is active during rest and activities like daydreaming, envisioning the future, and reflecting on the self. When we connect with others, oxytocin, also known as the love hormone and associated with bonding and emotional regulation, can be activated. When we connect with people we love or trust, oxytocin is released, helping us feel seen, loved, and supported. This can trigger dopamine, a neurotransmitter linked to reward and motivation, and it also plays a role in the creative process. Dopamine might be triggered by you saying *yes* to play, which results in the reward of fun, connection, joy, and feeling seen.

Imagine this: You plan a creative vision board date with your friends, where you laugh, eat, and connect, being present and enjoying the experience. That's a potential positive for oxytocin, DMN, and dopamine. All of these could potentially be aligned and powered on for your benefit.

What does this mean for you? When you say yes to play, joy, excitement, creativity, feeling alive, feeling satisfied, and to your well-being, you also say yes to your purpose.

A purposeful life isn't about winning the societally acceptable paths, and it's not about winning the fights that life throws your way. Feeling purposeful and believing you have a meaningful life comes from engaging in activities that feel supportive and inspiring too.

Like I mentioned earlier, people often think you're in a "crisis" when you decide to change your life drastically by introducing more play. Even the mere idea of entertaining yourself makes people want to "check your temperature" and see if you're okay; that's how starved of enjoyment our culture and communities are. The idea that you'd want to center fun in your life must mean you've lost your mind.

Time can't continue to be the reason you say no to yourself. And you can't continue to be the reason you say no to yourself. This is an opportunity for a curious play date with Little You. And maybe, invite your friends' Little Yous too. Join a local chorus. Rent a bicycle to run errands. Make mocktails with flavors you've never tried. Go on group afternoon walks. Host a dinner where guests help each other with their dream résumés. There are so many ways to have a play date with Little You.

Play helps you take a break from the rinse-and-repeat cycle that you've been taught is life. Yes, you may have days that feel like a fight, but your evenings can be your play dates. If you have kids or you're a caretaker, it's tougher to find time, so if you can, try to include them as much as possible. Sometimes I switch on my music, grab my kids, and dance for thirty minutes, even though I could be doing something else. I let Little Yas be with them. It might not be something you feel you can do all the time, but even if it's only once a week, you'll have something to look forward to. We need things to look forward to.

If I asked you to look back and name what you've healed, you'd probably list the relationships you cut off, your wellness regimen, and the village you built. You'd share what you stopped letting bother you, and you'd go on about the practices that changed the way you look at yourself and the world. You'd own that you were responsible for the beautiful changes that shifted you. You'd bask in the experience of people who know you, not recognizing this new energy that's washed over your entire being. And you'd delight in this because it strokes the ego part of you that says, *yes, I did a great thing. I mastered healing too.*

But honey, healing is forever. Celebrate the hard work you've done to master the art of choosing yourself, but be willing to name the ways you're still in your way. Being able to share the list of things you've healed is important but it's not why we're doing this work. The only "prize" we're after is living a fuller life.

Also, when you named the things that you've healed, did you also name joy? Is joy part of your life again? Don't get caught up thinking you're finished. Remember, there's no checklist, and we keep choosing ourselves again and again.

When I ask if *you're the reason you're unhappy,* I'm inviting you to consider how you might be partly responsible, and responsibility isn't sexy; I get that. We want to talk about all we *did* do. But responsibility is also part of purpose. Accountability helps you remember what matters. There's a shedding and then a reclamation.

Once you own the parts that are yours, you head directly to the pathway you desire.

> ### Get Curious
>
> How are you still saying yes to the rinse-and-repeat cycles that aren't working? How can you say yes to something new?

Remember, we're here to practice. I'm not here to fight you. I'm the one outside of the ring with a towel, water, and snacks. I have a strategy to help you win. I'm here to let you know, the fight is done for now. You've won this round.

> ### *Come Back to Yourself*
>
> Access the voicenotes section of your phone, hit record, and while you wash your face, say out loud the reasons it stings a little bit to be in the way of your happiness. Share how it doesn't feel fair, share how you disagree with this, share how you want to move forward, and share what it would take for you to try something new.

this is the era,
you stop telling yourself
you should be over it by now
in this era, you get to be witnessed.
you get to be celebrated.
you get to be held.
you get to be seen.
maybe your soul has been waiting on that.
for you to say the fight is over,
look out into the crowd,
and see that people aren't laughing,
they're rooting for you.
that's what you've been waiting for.

5 Have You Abandoned Parts of Yourself to Fit In?

Authenticity is hard to fake.

You can tell when someone's laugh is genuine, and whether they're wearing what makes them feel good, not just fit in. We can see it, but we can feel it too. We're told to love ourselves regardless, but it's tough to love yourself when you've received messages that say the opposite. Faking it until you make it is a Band-Aid that asks you to ignore what you're struggling with, and it's unhealthy if carried out long-term. Facing your struggles allows you to learn how to accept the beauty of who you are while making room to still become who you want to be.

Little You discarded the parts of you that were bullied, shamed, or seen as too much, out of absolute love for yourself. They didn't know how to find new friends or let the hurtful comments roll off, so Little You decided to bury the parts that didn't fit with others. Those parts may be hidden so deeply that you forgot where you placed them. But the transformation you're seeking will require you to reclaim them. You'll have to create spaces where it's okay to be your unique self, even if someone else thinks it's weird. I always tell my kids, "I'm so grateful that I'm a weird, creative, and silly person. It's a gift to be weird and wear it with pride."

And in case your skin prickled at the thought of owning weirdness, here are some of the synonyms of being weird: "unreal," "mysterious," "uncanny," and "supernatural." The opposite of weird? "Normal," "ordinary," and "conventional." You choose.

Deesha has an impressive résumé, but what shines most is her heart. You would never know that she worked in the most powerful building in the US because she is so incredibly humble. When I forget who I am and doubt creeps in, she is the first person to remind me of what I'm capable of. This is no surprise because she speaks globally about imposter syndrome, and I can't think of a better person to focus on here because her story highlights how she had to believe in herself despite the noise around her.

While I was talking with Deesha, she shared:

Deesha: I was always told that I was loud and it was never in a positive sense. I think I developed a voice very early out of rebellion because I was told so many times how bad I was for having a voice, and began to lean into that, and I'm still that way. The White House was oil, and I was water. When I stepped into that space as the White

House social secretary, I didn't know how to mix with it. And then I felt, I don't know if I want to mix with this, especially after I discovered it a bit more.

The Obamas hired me strictly on who I was and what they saw. So, what would it look like changing it up after six years with them? I knew being myself meant that I was going to be excluded. I knew that I would be talked about. I knew that it would be like, "Here comes Deesha." I knew all those things, and I had to accept the loneliness that comes with it. I knew the role was temporary because we had a finite date in the White House. So, I thought, I can either change myself and then have to do all that unchanging once I get out of here; I can change myself and then not recognize myself at all; or I could be me.

And I didn't decide this on purpose. When the naysayers started talking, it hurt but I also thought, *well, Barack and Michelle Obama appointed me to this position, and you don't matter.* I didn't realize what an asset not changing was until now, when people come up to me and say, "Deesha, the way you did that in the White House, you taught us to be ourselves." And now I'm like, oh, I was brave.

Getting to know the parts of you that were hidden might feel hard at first, but fight for them to exist. Whatever parts you thought you had to leave behind, let's collect them—your humor, silliness, grit, ruggedness, strength, forgetfulness—you. You never have to be what the world has decided was *cool* ever again.

The peer pressure that exists, even as an adult, is in the way of your purpose. It's time to let that go and be free.

Get Curious

Imagine for a moment that you only had supportive people around you. They share the truth when necessary, but they want to see you win. They love you wholeheartedly. What would you do with that kind of support? Where would you live? Who would you date? What would you admit? You may not have this supportive circle yet, but you can move toward the life you want as if it exists.

By using this imaginative space, you'll connect with what you want and the stories, beliefs, or limitations that hold you back from it.

Yes, things would be easier if you had help, then and now. But what if you are the only person who can save you?

By reclaiming the parts that Little You hid away, you become the hero and save **yourself**; it's impossible to *hide* and *be seen*. It's time to step out. People will continue to share unsolicited opinions and feedback about who they think you are, but if you don't believe it, it doesn't have to stop you.

During the past ten years, I've encouraged thousands of people to write letters to themselves. When you talk directly to yourself, you open channels of communication that you probably didn't think were possible. You bring the keys of wisdom right to the locks.

To reunite with the parts of you that didn't feel safe living out loud, I wrote to our collective selves below. Some of this won't feel relatable, and some might feel like I'm speaking directly to you. Keep what's for you and release what isn't.

To "The You" Afraid of Being Judged:
You had good reason to be afraid of being negatively critiqued because you've watched people get torn apart with no regard for how it left them feeling. You never wanted to be in the middle of those who gathered to see your expression when their hurtful words pierced your heart. So, you stuffed away your light, magic, and freeness, hoping it would protect you. The shame you felt never came from not loving your gifts; it came from loving who you are so much that you thought keeping yourself safe meant not expressing yourself out loud.

Remember, you're safe, and it's time to live out loud.

To "The You" with Expectations:
When you became brave enough to be yourself and you weren't met with the response you hoped for, your expectations were lowered—almost completely erased. Even when you allowed yourself to have expectations of those who were supposed to be *your people*, you learned quickly that sometimes even those who say they love you can't always handle your shine. *It reminds them of what they haven't said yes to for themselves.* Maybe they're happy for you, but don't show it in a way that helps you feel it. Perhaps they want you to be a light, but within their limits. Your willingness to stand as you are threatens their fears and beliefs, so they ask you to stay small by ignoring your bigness. They ignore it so well, you don't believe it's there. They need you to adhere to all the made-up rules, so they don't have to get uncomfortable. This was never your work, and yet somehow it became your responsibility to keep yourself in line.

You learned it was safer to do away with expectations and count on people disappointing you. Even yourself. This was a way to control your feelings and not experience the shock of being let down. By attempting to keep yourself from being disappointed, you kept out the good too.

Remember, it's safe to let the good in because people are waiting to love you.

To "The You" that You Are with Everyone Else:

Part of you feels like you've given up so much time in the name of protecting yourself that you aren't interested in changing anything else at this point, even if it means coming back to your true self. You've accepted that you are who everyone else says you are, even if it's completely made up. You know what outfits people will respond to, you know which dishes people like that you make, and you know what people want from you. You've gotten *good* at being that person for them.

When you try something new and share it, only to have people respond with a tone that suggests *it's not something you'd ever do,* you tend to believe them. Why wouldn't you? They're a mirror of who you are, right? It isn't until you decide that you're the one that reflects the truth that you'll truly shine as you were intended to.

Remember, it's safe to be who you say you are.

To "The You" who Was Blamed + Shamed:

Sometimes being ourselves means we say or do things that get us in trouble, and it's usually our little selves who pay the price. Even though we were young, we received a response meant for an adult (or for no one), and we've held the weight of those experiences that were far too heavy to carry. It didn't help us build resilience; it made us afraid. We learned right then and there: Being curious, inquisitive, or *too clever for our own good* is dangerous. Therefore, any part of us that appears to be different is tucked away. Of course, we think we'll go back for it, but then life happens, and we get distracted.

When purpose still seems like some faraway thing that we're all trying to reach for an unknown reason, many of us are trying to determine *what it's all for.* I won't pretend that I have the answers, however, I can share my belief. *I believe you were born at this time to bring exactly what you have to the world.* I believe the world needs your gifts for the time that you're here. I wish we didn't have to fight to stay connected to who we are, but remember, in the fight, Little You will always be on your side.

We don't often think about betrayal when we think about fitting in, but at some point, someone we felt we could trust showed us even those who love us can let us down. Maybe they talked about you behind your back or said hurtful things to your face. Perhaps they behaved as if they didn't know you or made fun of you for the very reasons you thought they loved you. When Little You experienced betrayal, they set up systems within to ensure it would never happen again. Unfortunately, Little You didn't know these systems of "protection" would encourage you to betray yourself because those very systems abandon who you are. Whether this shows up in friendships, romantic relationships, at work, or with yourself, we have all, at some point, abandoned parts of ourselves for the sake of safety. It's time to make room for those parts to exist again.

Your people will make it easy to choose to let those buried parts be free. Your new hair, career, or flair will be celebrated. Your new ideas and excitement will be met with

"Tell me more" and *"I'd love to explore them with you!"* Some relationships won't fit your whole self, but it's also true that some will grow beyond what you believed possible now that you've said yes to holding all of you. This is an essential part of building your **community**: knowing what works and what doesn't.

When you show up with your abandoned parts, and you genuinely connect with someone, without any armor, you've found *belonging*. This person speaks your energetic language, and it should feel *easy*. As your connection grows, they'll be willing to walk with you even when you don't know where you want to go. They want the best for you without believing it's their responsibility to choose the direction you go. They know you but don't pretend to know you better than you know yourself. They're just happy to be with you.

Chloe embodies bringing all parts of you to the table in such a beautiful way. When you walk into her home, you'll see a stunning canvas of art she's painting, remnants of the writer's dinner she hosted the night before, and as you sit down, she'll tell you about the retreat in Greece that's happening in six months. She does all this while making her friends feel seen and loved, and while also working a nine-to-five career that requires focus on significant, purpose-driven work.

While I was talking to Chloe, she shared:

Chloe: I want to be more strategic in my creative career, and there are things that I just want to do because I've always wanted to. I don't need to do it multiple times, but I want to have an art exhibit. I want to do a one-woman monologue show. I went to a clairvoyant over the summer, and she said, "You are in a stage in your life where you are more childlike than you ever were because when you were a child, you had to grow up very fast and you couldn't afford to be a child in the way that you should have been. So now that you're at this age, you're experimenting. You're allowing life to be more of a playground."

I think it's beautiful and healing to want to do these things that are so random, that are really not random because they're so much a part of you. They just haven't been let outside the closet.

When you said no to your bravest, chicest, most spectacular self, you also said no to the things that light you up. It's one thing to say, I'm not ready to write a book, but I'm going to keep researching, growing in confidence, and playing with storytelling until I feel ready. Yes, you aren't writing the book yet, but you're still working toward it. It's living in you and the world.

It's a very different thing to use the negative feedback you received on your writing as evidence not to move forward, abandoning a dream that can become stronger with practice. When you decide to never speak of writing again, you hide that part of you as a protection mechanism. But once it's hidden, it's out of your sight. So, you're not protected; it's keeping you from your gifts.

Your purpose-driven life needs your off-the-wall ideas, originality, creativity, your beliefs, experience, and your natural ability to convey your gift like no one else can. Being connected to your whole self is what helps you feel worthy. Your worthiness enables you to pursue what you desire.

Our worthiness is the very thing that helps us love ourselves and others, because it frees us from judgment and expectation. When you know you're unconditionally loved, you allow yourself to be seen.

For me, Little Yas at the ages of twelve, fifteen, sixteen, and nineteen usually comes to mind. They were critical coming-of-age moments that I still reflect on, where I made decisions that changed how I saw myself. My first move and starting over in a different neighborhood, the first boyfriend, and the decision to leave home at nineteen. Life-changing moments.

If you feel those parts of you come up with a lot to get off their chest, while doing any other task—while you're showering, washing your face, etc.—say Little You's words out loud. Speaking Little You's truth helps you show love to those quiet parts of you. And don't worry if you're taking a walk in public while doing this; pretend you're on a phone call. No one will know you're talking to your younger self. What would twelve-year-old you say if they had the freedom to speak?

What would you have said in your twenties if you felt safe enough to admit it?

What would you have told your parents? What would you have told your friends? Who did you want to hang out with that you were afraid wasn't cool? Who would you have broken up with?

Allow them to tell you what they think about your life now. Even if you forgot those parts of you existed, they've never forgotten about you. Where do they wish you would be less afraid? What do they wish you said yes to? How are they hoping to contribute to the meaningful life you're building for yourself? Let Little You share the parts of your life they're proud of too.

You won't reclaim those parts of yourself by doing a ten-step routine, meditating every day, eating right, cold plunging, or getting in enough steps. These things will help your mind and body, but that's not the way toward your purpose.

You reclaim those parts that Little You hid to keep you safe by doing what they were never allowed to do before: letting them speak. Open the door of communication that was pushed away from the forefront of your mind. You'll be amazed at what they have to say to you.

> ### Come Back to Yourself
> This week, while doing adulting tasks (like laundry), think about what your purpose means to those little parts of you reclaimed in this chapter. Ask yourself, am I ready to allow my whole self to make new rules?

We've journeyed through curiosity together, and I hope it's given you space to reconnect with Little You, so that you hold closely who you are at your core. We're always trying to give that part of us what they never had or what we had at one time that's shifted. But it's time for a change. Your curiosity will continue to open doors, but as you move forward, it's time to give structure to this moment of awakening, so with each small step, you feel steady. It's time. Keep going. Your comeback is in motion.

in this era,
you're brave enough
to remember
who you've always been . . .
and come back home to you.

PART II

Remembering

W ITH CURIOUS EYES AND MINDS, WE searched for ourselves. And that curiosity has brought us to a place of deep familiarity. Why does it feel safe to explore your soul? Why does it feel safe to learn what's changed within? Why does it feel safe to discover more about you?

Because you're remembering.

Your life is waiting, and it's patient. It won't judge you; it doesn't care how long it takes.

You've arrived exactly when you were supposed to. It's not too late.

Bring your light and know that with every step you take, no matter how small, you grow.

To remembering.

6 The Seven C's of Purpose

Water is a healer.

It reminds us to go with the flow, surrender to the unexpected, and be restored beyond our control. When I noticed that the seven guiding principles I'm about to share all start with the letter "C," I was reminded of the *seven seas,* and I thought, it's kismet that these have a framework similar to these powerful bodies of water.

I created the Seven C's to help you establish a deep connection with your purpose and to surrender your old programming. Remembering who you are opens the door to transformational healing.

The number seven holds meaning for many, including myself. In Hinduism, there are seven chakras. In Christianity, there are the seven days of creation. In Islam, there are seven heavens mentioned in the Quran. Judaism has seven branches of the menorah. The Buddha took seven steps at birth, symbolizing his path to enlightenment and representing the seven directions of the Universe. Japanese culture has the Seven Lucky Gods. And we all know, even if we've never hit the slots ourselves, how the number seven is revered as fortunate in gambling.

There are seven colors in the rainbow, seven musical notes before they are all repeated in the next octave, seven days of the week, seven continents, and seven wonders of the world.

Seven feels sacred. The Seven C's help us define purpose for ourselves, noting that, collectively, we have an idea of what purpose *means;* yet, individually, we might need purpose to mean something completely different.

I hope you continue to cultivate curiosity as you define or refine your purpose, and I hope these seven guiding principles help you assess what that purpose means to you. Everything you do in the world won't be meaningful, and that's okay, but if you're devoting a significant amount of time or energy toward something, it should significantly matter.

Keep these Seven C's close. Notice which ones are the most challenging to listen to and pay attention to what you feel in your body. Our bodies often know the truth before we're willing to acknowledge it in our brains.

The Seven C's aren't rules, but they'll help you be honest with yourself about things you'd usually ignore—like the job you can't stand, the lack of a real community around you, the happiness you're missing each morning, etc. These C's act as a litmus test as you learn to trust your intuition again. If something in your life hits each of the C's, it's probably significant. It doesn't mean you won't have challenging human experiences or go through hard times. It doesn't mean you won't struggle.

The Seven C's were created as a guide to help that internal part of you clouded by internal chatter, fears, and worries . . . but they aren't a concrete solution. There will be times when one of these principles feels incredibly important, and other times in your life when you completely shift focus. Let there be nuance. Allow yourself to change your mind. The most beautiful thing you can offer your purpose is freedom. That's kind of what we say yes to when we say yes to our purpose anyway. We're saying we're willing to be led, we're willing to surrender, and we're willing to go in a new direction even when we don't know where we'll arrive. Purpose is an invitation to trust.

The beauty of the Seven C's is that they're here to help you call your power within yourself and answer the hard questions.

Remember, you get to choose.

THE SEVEN C'S
1. Commitment

When you're devoted to something, you wake up feeling excited about what you get to do. Even when you're tired, when life is tough, or when you're down, your commitments are the things that keep you going. When you don't want to keep going, commitment is the *why* that encourages you to say yes anyway. **Commitment offers you something bigger than yourself.**

Keeping promises to yourself is a trust-building exercise like no other. There's no gentle way to say this, but having good intentions is not enough. You need to be willing to do exactly what you say you're going to do for yourself. The caveat is if you say you're going to write at five a.m. but sleep in and don't wake up until eight a.m., and still manage to complete your writing, you've still shown up. You don't need perfection. You do need space for flow. **You definitely need commitment.**

When you disregard what you said you would do because it's uncomfortable, you will remain uncomfortable. Your purpose will continue to feel unreachable. **The story you tell yourself about it not being possible will only be true because you say it is, through your inaction.**

Commitment is a choice, and you have to *want* it. Your purpose is allowed to change, but your willingness to commit must be grounded in reality. If you don't want it, it's not for you.

> ### Ask Yourself
>
> Am I committed to this? Am I willing to try again if it fails? Am I willing to admit I'm not the most experienced in the room, and am I willing to not let that hold me back? Am I willing to be a small part of significant change if it leads toward the goal? Am I willing to work hard for this? What am I willing to sacrifice to have this?

This "C" is nonnegotiable. If you feel strongly about something you're here to do, you must commit to working toward it. If you struggle with commitment, you must commit to working on what keeps you from committing so you can show up. There is no way around this one, and that's tough because commitment is hard.

Commitment can't be faked. Be real with yourself and don't try to "make it work." Instead, ask yourself why this isn't working, and take the steps to change it, because when it's a yes, it'll fit like a glove. To practice committing, find ways to connect what you love doing with what you don't. Hate doing laundry but love listening to podcasts? Combine them. Struggling with writer's block, but you want to write a book? Set a time limit for how long you will write, and sit there playing your favorite music for the whole duration, even if no words come to mind. Show up no matter what. When you learn this trick, you can commit even when it's tough, and you'll discover you don't have to lose yourself or the things that light you up just because it's hard.

Example: *When Lia started her anonymous blog, she was **committing** to the writing she'd always wanted to do. This small commitment eventually led her to write for popular publications and host her own podcast. The small commitments can become big things.*

> ### Affirmation
>
> I'm committed to myself and will continue to show up because I matter.

2. Community

Community helps you feel seen, supported, and loved. It inspires you, roots for you, and keeps you company. If you don't feel like you have meaning in your life, it might be because you lack meaningful relationships with people you see regularly. Connection is an integral part of purpose.

If you have good people around you but intentionally avoid them, it might be because, unconsciously, you know they will reflect the things that are wrong in your life. When you don't have a community around, you can *keep living the lie*. Good friends will not silently watch you make terrible choices.

If you find yourself alienating the people around you, ask yourself if you're stepping back into your cycle of secrets. Ask yourself if you're afraid of being hurt. Ask yourself if this is helping you.

When you say yes to a new community, look at who you've said yes to. The people around you don't need to be perfect; we all have people in our lives who aren't committed to themselves in the best way, but that's their responsibility. We can love them and still be part of their lives. However, if you're committed to building a new life for yourself and the community around you doesn't align with your goals, you'll be distracted. Choose yourself and surround yourself with a community who can support you.

This "C" is incredibly valuable. People who have a community might lack the other C's, but they can find their sense of worth and purpose within the community they belong to. Relationships and the way we're seen and loved help us remember that we belong. The world can throw complicated things your way, and you will still stand because you have people willing to stand hand in hand with you.

> ### — *Ask Yourself* —
>
> Do I lean into my community? Have I leaned toward solo work versus community work because of past negative experiences in my community? Is building a new community a scary or intimidating experience? What does community mean to me?

Example: *Deesha found herself in an environment at the White House that initially felt incompatible with who she was.*

But rather than conforming, she leaned into her true self and allowed her community to reflect her, eventually becoming a role model for others to do the same.

— *Affirmation* —

I always belong exactly as I am.

3. Creativity

Creativity is not about starting a side hustle or business, and it's not about using your gifts solely to please others. It's about living a life where your creations leave you delighted at seeing the ideas you dreamed of come to life.

If you've been micromanaged, shamed, talked down to, ignored, told to stay in your lane, or overlooked, it probably impacted your creative expression. Do past experiences hinder your creativity? Have you been able to prioritize creativity in your life?

Creativity isn't something most of us make space for daily unless we create for a living. As an author and paid creative, I also know that if you're not careful, your precious gifts can be stalled by feedback, production, and deadlines. In other words, if you don't make space to create outside of what you're paid to do, you can lose the fun.

Deep down, we're all creators. We all view the world uniquely. Creativity grants freedom. Having a meaningful life requires embracing creativity beyond merely absorbing what others make.

The work you do might be creative, like being an electrician, chef, teacher, or construction worker, and if it scratches the itch of imagination and innovation for you, that's amazing. You don't have to re-create the wheel if you genuinely feel you are creating something new every day through your work. But your life is driven by the way you choose to live it, so ensure that it isn't always about work; it's also for you.

This "C" might be part of your life already in sneaky ways: the way you cook, dress, style your hair, or encourage others. Make this as easy on yourself as you can. Doodle, try new things, play, and allow inspiration to get you started.

> ### *Ask Yourself*
>
> How do I use my creativity in ways that I was un-aware of before? What do I think being creative means, and does it match my truth? If I could do something creative, what would it be? What did Little Me enjoy doing creatively?

Example: *Chloe's desire to have an art exhibit honors a creative part of herself that hadn't "been let outside the closet." She's honoring her dreams even though they're separate from her career, and that's fueling her.*

> ### *Affirmation*
>
> I was born a creator and have been innovating my whole life. Creating will always be part of me, and it's safe to bring it into everything I do.

4. Compelling

Most of the things you commit to in your life need to be compelling. You should feel inspired, interested, and fascinated, even if you've been doing it for years. When you're not inspired by what you've said yes to, it's bound to impact *how* you show up.

It's not about how shiny it is or how shiny it makes you look. The luster only lasts for a little while. Even the excitement of the pay bump is short-lived. There's a popular saying, "Choose a job you love, and you'll never work a day in your life." Enjoyable work is indeed easier to look forward to, but you're still working. The sooner we separate *work* from what we do for ourselves, the better.

What are the compelling interests that keep you feeling connected to Little You? When you say yes to things that connect to your younger self, you'll look forward to them even when you're overwhelmed and when life is tough. You'll still crave the art, relationships, and volunteering when it's time to adult. If it fills you up to be a mentor in your community, you'll show up even when you're in the middle of a storm. You'll still honor your meditation practice with a full schedule, because you know saying yes to yourself feels good. You'll keep showing up because you're inspired and you believe in it.

This "C" is where you'll find your true sense of self. What inspires you is unique to you, and the willingness to follow the invitation of inspiration will keep you aligned with what matters to you.

Ask Yourself

Am I spending my time on things that inspire me? Or is the majority of my time spent on what I think I have to do?

Example: *What truly compelled Amanda, despite the success and status of her previous career, was the work in healing and spirituality that she always thought would be a hobby. Her small steps over the years helped her stay inspired and ultimately changed the trajectory of her professional path and life.*

— Affirmation —

I listen when inspiration speaks to me, and I trust it will lead me where I need to be.

---

5. Choice

Is your life a reflection of what you want? Or is your life a reflection of circumstances that feel as if they've happened outside of your control? Of course, you may be creating and working in areas that your family or friends have led you to, but your decision to commit to them should have been yours. Your devotion to them should be your choice, not a jail sentence.

I recognize that many of us have serious commitments that, in hindsight, don't feel like something we would say yes to again. Kids, marriages, careers, degrees, tattoos. There are so many "choices" that at the time, we didn't have enough information to make the best decision. It's hard because now we feel stuck with the commitment.

Remember, choosing and commitment are linked, but they're not the same. Some choices leave us with obligations we can't undo. Some options are hard to commit to. Some commitments were never our choice.

In the future, I want you to say "yes" and "no" as confidently as you can. Confidently change your mind. Be the boss and make decisions. Removing the repetitive and tedious aspects of your life will require you to **do something, to choose something.** You can't expect change without choosing something different. It must come from you, or time will feel like it's passing you by. Just look back at your life if you don't believe me! It will not change without you!

This "C" leads with empowerment. You get to choose. Whether you're married, a parent, or have a career, there's no limit. Even if you've never danced but want to take salsa lessons. Even if you want to be on Broadway, but you're forty-five and think time has passed you by. The only limits that exist are the ones you honor as if they're real.

> ### Ask Yourself
> I now have the chance to choose anything, so what will it be? What do I choose?

Example: *Amanda's choice to set boundaries when she returned to New York after her sabbatical demonstrated the power of choosing yourself. She said, "I realized, wow, they still like and respect me" even with hard boundaries. This life-changing realization helped her continue to prioritize herself as she moved on in her career and life.*

> ### Affirmation
> I'm in the power position when I remember that I get to choose.

6. Confirming

You'll know you're living in alignment when *the choices you've made confirm things about yourself that you wouldn't have known if you didn't say yes.* What does this mean? You will discover who you are by committing to what you want and allowing that unfolding to reveal beautiful aspects of yourself that were previously unknown. You may feel like *I didn't know I was capable of that,* but you always were. And what's even more inspiring is others will see the changes in you too. Saying yes to what feels like a divine assignment will give you a different energy. It will radiate through you.

Some new parents share that *their child has given them purpose because they finally feel like they're doing what they're here to do.* Some people devote their lives to traveling the world, immersing themselves in different cultures, and each time they land in a new place, they *feel like they're exactly where they're meant to be.* Whether you feel called to start a lifestyle blog, teach people a new language, volunteer at a shelter, or learn to make pottery, when what you do is a **yes,** it will confirm a truth within you, and you will feel it. And others will see it.

Your life will be filled with moments that shape who you're becoming, but we can't always live for what we're planning in the future. Enjoy the present too.

> ### Ask Yourself
>
> How is what I've filled my life with validating the way I want to live? Are my projects, creations, relationships, or my work a reflection of what matters deeply to me?

This "C" is an opportunity for reflection. Your past fears of what others think, who you're "supposed" to be, and what you want applause for will show up. You've said yes to draining things to confirm false truths in the eyes of the people you wanted to make proud. But your people pleaser self can be laid to rest. You can decide to choose you > everything.

Example: *When Britt attended a circus show featuring everyday people, she received confirmation that it wasn't too late for her dream. There were people out there just like her—people who did one thing professionally but were interested in the same things she was—and it was brave to go after what you want, no matter what people think.*

> **Affirmation**
>
> My life reflects what matters to me.

7. Challenging

Maybe you didn't expect to see this word here, but it's essential. If you're not feeling challenged, what once felt shiny and new will eventually feel like Groundhog Day: the same thing, a different day. Rinse and repeat. I know this challenges the beliefs we have about a well-lived life. You might be telling yourself that your life needs to feel *easier* or *less complicated* so you can have more fun. That's true when it comes to drama-filled relationships, demanding jobs with no passion, and many of the other areas we touched on earlier.

However, being challenged in a healthy way helps you stay committed, encourages you to lean on your community, inspires you to use your creativity, and keeps you interested. It must be something you choose every day, otherwise it won't work. It's the reason this "C" is last, because you need the other "C's" for this "C" to feel good. Otherwise, it's just a challenge with no meaning, no inspiration, and no choice.

It's exciting to start a new project *you've worked hard on*, watch it grow, and gain buy-in. It's exhilarating to *put your work out there* and discover people are interested and touched by what you do. It's rewarding to build a team. It's inspiring to try pottery for the first time. It's powerful to wear the monochromatic pink suit to the work meeting where everyone else will be in black or blue. It's gratifying to send the pitch email. It's beautifully humbling to be met by your friends when you share vulnerably.

All these positive experiences are met with **a challenge at first**. It was a risk to put your whole self out there and potentially not be received the way you expected. Believe it or not, this "C" is what keeps you going. You'll learn your lessons here, grow here, and build wisdom here. You get brave and decide to pick yourself up when it doesn't work out here. Your resilience, stamina, and confidence are built here.

You will thrive here.

> ### — *Ask Yourself* —
>
> How have I been running from challenges because, frankly, I'm tired? How can I redefine challenges as a positive motivator that I've used in the past to thrive?

Example: *Britt, Lia, Chloe, Deesha, and Amanda committed themselves to living in a way that feels good but still challenges them. Britt is challenged through her performances, Amanda is challenged in her spiritual practice, Chloe is challenged by finding new ways to express her creativity, Deesha is challenged through exploring joy in new ways, and Lia is challenged to tell her story through her writing journey. Even if the challenge they've named feels easy to you, for them it's a risk, a big step, and the same goes for you. We, individually, name our challenge and decide what it means to us.*

Affirmation

In the face of challenges, I continue to thrive.

Remember, the Seven C's is a guide that steers you into your comeback era. This is the era where you walk boldly with the wisdom, encouragement, support, and guidance you've always desired. It's going to come from within you and from around you. Keep going.

Note: Throughout the rest of the book, Seven C words that directly connect you to your purpose, your meaningful life, or what matters to you will be **bold**. These are foot-stomping, hard-hitting, finger-snapping reminders. Read those sentences twice if you need to.

7 What Did Little You Want to Be When You Grew Up?

Remember what it felt like to be asked, "What do you want to be when you grow up?"

It was exciting to dream about what your life could be, share your ideas, and be met with genuine interest. If you wanted to be a doctor, everyone smiled along with you. No one got technical about the qualifications or brought up your struggles. If you wanted to be a math teacher, everyone delighted in your desire. And if you mentioned being a firefighter because you want to help people, there were oohs and aahs. You received validation and smiles because you were brave enough to say what you wanted out loud.

As you grew, the question became harder to answer, and the pressure increased. It was clear that the same people who delighted in your dreams now expected something more.

What was your plan? When were you going to start being *realistic*? Many adults say, *I'm still trying to figure out what I want to be when I grow up*, which always reminds me that no matter how old you get, there's always this sense you're *still growing up*.

We've discussed the pressure we feel to obtain degrees, accept jobs, and say yes to opportunities that don't align with who we are but instead with what the world expects us to be. However, we haven't discussed people who choose careers where their work is centered on impacting a community. No matter what we do, we all have an impact. However, these roles, often thought of as "purpose-driven," are typically in service jobs, such as nursing, nonprofit work, organizing, teaching, or those in companies that support industries directly benefiting people.

It's essential to note that many purpose-driven jobs don't offer a large salary, if one is received at all, but they exist because people are driven by their desire to serve. Volunteers at soup kitchens and animal shelters, Girl Scout troop leaders, and youth coaches are roles typically filled by people who want to support others, regardless of the sacrifices they may face.

While I was chatting with Chloe about purpose, she shared:

I can honestly say that in my seventeen-year career, paying my bills hasn't been my priority. I've always needed purpose-driven work. My mother arrived in Niger when she was twenty years old in the seventies. She had me and raised me as a single mother, a single white woman raising a brown child in Africa. I was exposed to the divide of privilege and lack of access very early, and my mom's work was in global development. Her work wasn't in a fancy office; it took her into very remote places. She oversaw nursing programs, agricultural programs, and youth programs. Her work was literally saving lives. I appreciated that. One thing my mom always taught me just by example is there's dignity in everyone, in every discipline, and everybody's story.

I love this story from Chloe because it shows how our **commitment** to our work can stem from people or moments throughout our lives that we've found meaningful. Commitment is one of the hardest of the Seven C's, because life often gets in the way of consistency. But magic happens when you find a way to weave your story and what matters to you into your commitment.

The words you use to describe yourself matter. Do you carry your story with dignity, or is that an area needing love and attention from you? Whether it's how you survived against all odds or how you had the village of a lifetime rooting for you every step of the way, all of these stories impacted what you thought was possible, even at a very young age. Your stories helped shape who you wanted to become as you grew.

So, when I ask you, "What did Little You want to be?" I hope early on, you had a very self-serving answer. I hope it was something **you** wanted, and not what you thought you had to say because of what people wanted to hear. Or, if you felt pressure to be what everyone needed you to be, I hope you find the courage to admit now what you've always known to be true. Lia always knew that writing was what she wanted, but she chose a career that *felt like the right fit at the time, especially for others.* The good news? Lia reclaimed what she loves, and she's been writing for some time now. Lia shared:

> I have about forty-five journals from childhood. When I go back to my journals, it's always the evidence of what I was feeling and thinking. Because when I see myself in photos, I can't quite remember clearly what I felt in that moment as I toggle between the story I told the world versus what was my real story. So, my childhood journals not only corroborate that I wanted to be a writer, but they were also my vessels for the truth.
>
> When I started to work through my own mental health issues, the first thing I did was start an anonymous blog. Now I'm at a place where I want to talk about my broken vagina on a podcast I host. So, it's just interesting to see how that calling or that draw was like a secret, and I kept the desire to be a writer as something private, whereas now I'm just much more open about wanting to tell the truth. In my childhood, there was so much confusion about what the truth was in my household. So, I had to go on this journey to try to uncover that.

As much as I've preached about purpose being more than just what you do, how we earn a living does matter. Some people have an unfulfilling job, but they've made peace with it because it funds everything that matters to them. Some have a job that doesn't pay much, but the work fills them up. It's not easy, but it's possible to have both fulfillment and the pay you need.

Every single person I interviewed lit up when I asked them what they wanted to be when they were growing up. Talking about their dreams from the perspective of their little selves brought up memories that felt good. For some, once the memory was acknowledged, it was tough to witness because it no longer felt possible, but I want us to change that. Please use these memories to propel you forward, rather than keep you trapped in your past.

Imagine getting to do the seemingly outlandish things you dreamed of as a child, like discovering more about dinosaurs, digging for treasure, singing, vintage shopping, Lego collecting, or any other dream Little You had. What if they were accepted and supported by you? If you could choose right now, what would it be?

More importantly, what are you waiting for?

We now live in a world where people can start side hustles or creative outlets online. I've watched someone cook a luxurious meal over a wood-burning fire in the middle of the woods. I've watched people create beautiful, sprawling paintings using recycled cardboard. I've watched people buy two-dollar garments from fifty years before they were born and transform them into something that looks like it came straight off the runway. I don't know if these people are paid for what they share, but I know they're making what matters to them. They're creating from a purpose-driven place.

While researching, I considered the concept of purpose-driven work and how it provides meaning in people's lives, regardless of whether they are paid for it. *What would it look like if we took the word "work" and changed it to "life"?* What if everything in your life was driven by the things that matter most to you? What if saying yes to the part of you that wants more creates space for your **purpose-driven life?**

I discovered an incredible research perspective called the Serious Leisure Perspective, or SLP. SLP explores how people participate in activities or experiences that have nothing to do with their career but still contribute to their overall sense of fulfillment.[1]

SLP's principles include things like perseverance, personal effort, and career-like progression, but instead, you apply them toward things that have nothing to do with work. It encourages you to approach your Lego building with the same tenacity that you would use to achieve a promotion. It enables you to persevere when crocheting your first cardigan the same way you would through a challenge with a work project.

SLP activities include writing, creating art, volunteering, and engaging in a wide range of hobbies. When we wake up with something to do each day that isn't just about work or kids or others, it fulfills us and helps us feel satisfied with our lives. And we don't just *feel* satisfied, we **are satisfied.**

Creativity is essential because living is not just about what you do; it's also about who you are. We often downplay the importance of creativity and fail to discuss its impact on our well-being. Creativity is as essential as water and air.

How does this connect to what Little You wanted to be when you grew up, and ultimately, to a purpose-driven life?

It connects because you still hold those dreams that Little You had. You might not fulfill them exactly as you originally envisioned, but they're still waiting for you to say yes. If you have kids, nieces or nephews, or have spent time with children, you know they'll ask you to play about one thousand times. Each time you say no, their little voices get lower, and their heads drop lower too. Eventually, they stop asking, and it's because they no longer want to face disappointment. It doesn't mean they don't want to play with you; they no longer have the confidence to ask. This is precisely what happened between adult you and Little You.

When you tell your Little You "no" when they ask you to play or connect with yourself, you're saying *"yes, I agree what you're asking me to do is going to be fun,* **but** *no, I can't play today."* And when you do that repeatedly to yourself, that part of you gets tired of asking, and the voice and head drop lower and lower. Eventually, that part of you, Little You, becomes sick of the disappointment and stops asking.

> ——— *Remember for a Moment* ———
>
> What were you craving to try as a child, as a teen, as a young adult, or in your thirties or forties? What are you craving right now? Don't have time to write a book? Start with a short story. Don't think you're a good cook? Start by making a no-cook dip. Unsure on how to change your style? Mix and match the clothes you already own using outfits you love as inspiration. Afraid to try something new? Ask a friend to join you.

Lean into those Seven C's, especially **community**, **creativity**, and **commitment**, when it comes to this. Invite your **community** to join you, at least the first time. Start small, but choose something that will allow you to be flexible as you begin.

And now, try changing the story. When I asked, "What did you want to be when you grew up?" you had the story you've been telling a long time, but it probably didn't include the part where you still believed it could come true, and we're here to change that. Now you can tell a new story that's something like this:

I wanted to be ________________ when I grew up, but I ended up choosing different paths. For various reasons at the time, these paths seemed safer and felt like the right thing to do. In many ways, I chose the path I did because I received ______________, ______________, and ______________ by going that route.

I used to say, "It wasn't meant to be" as a way of making sense of what never came to fruition. But now I know, yes, it wasn't meant to be in the way I originally planned, but I can start now. Even if it doesn't pay the bills, if it makes me happy, I'm willing to try.

There's power in rewriting your stories and speaking your new story out loud. When you say yes to something new, you change your generational pattern. The stiff, stagnant energy that once lived there has been cleared out, making way for fresh, flowing energy to take its place. In grief, you can still say yes to play. In sadness, you can still say yes to play. In disappointment, you can still say yes to play. You are big enough, brave enough, and safe enough to hold space for all the little versions of you that come up to you and tap you gently with their big idea of what would be great to try. And if you say no, let it be because it's not for you, not because you've subscribed to believing those past stories that say it's too late.

I love Chloe's story of seeing her mom dedicate her life to purpose-driven work and how, through seeing it, she chose that kind of work for herself. She knew it was possible and went into adult life with a story that empowered her to help others through a meaningful career.

We don't always have the mentors or examples that we need, but let the little versions of you watch **grown-up you** today as you say yes to building your purpose-driven life. What if, in your childlike way, you stopped when something was no longer fun and tried something else without judgment, without attachment, and without defense? Just as you see a child put down a toy and pick up a new one with no attachment, deciding to play with what feels good in the moment can be a great way to practice. Little You already speaks this language, and knows what you want. You don't have to learn anything new.

What if you allowed yourself to feel excited the next time someone asked you what you'd been up to? What if you shared your joy, your project, *your thing* with the excitement and smile that you never had? Please share how you're learning to skateboard, paint portraits, act in a play, coach the cheerleading team at the community center, or whatever it is that you've said yes to that has nothing to do with your career.

And when people follow up with questions like *Wow, what made you start doing that?*, you'll get to answer with pride, rather than say blanket statements to cover the fact that you're scared to be excited in front of people who may judge you because of reasons that aren't your responsibility to figure out. You will share your excitement out loud—for you. If it's received with a weird reaction, this is not your work.

Children are used to hearing other kids scream out what they're excited about with no context, no meaning, and no reason. Childhood is an environment of oversharing joy until around middle school, when—all of a sudden—it's not cool to enjoy yourself out loud anymore. It may have been months since the adult you're talking to has heard someone say they're doing something that genuinely excites them. No sarcasm, no joke, just excitement. They'll be standing in your light, and if you haven't been in your light in a while, you'll look different. It'll be like they're talking to a new person.

And the truth is they are. It's an embodied you. A you that's come back in the best way, remembering all those lost parts and bringing them back together, without needing to fix or control, and allowing yourself to be. Standing in your light will either free some people or scare them away. This makes owning your light **challenging** because experiencing other people's responses isn't always easy. This isn't your responsibility. Continue to be honest, creative, and live your purpose-driven life.

Come Back to Yourself

Get your phone, head to the notes app, and type out five things that you've always wanted to try that are within your means to do. Get creative. It can be anything that excites you. Now envision what it would be like to do the one you're most excited to try. Maybe while you're doing the dishes tonight, or getting yourself ready for bed, think about this thing that gives you childlike joy. Perhaps it's what Little You wanted to be or maybe not. Either way, it's your choice. Have fun, you get to choose.

P.S. You don't have to take any action or make any plans yet. Just allow your imagination to flourish.

i pray
your life
looks like something
you dreamed.
i pray you
look in the mirror
and barely recognize
yourself
because
you're overflowing
with joy.

8 Do You Want What You've Worked For?

Imagine, for a moment, all the time you've spent worrying, praying, and dreaming has paid its dues, and now you're rewarded. The time you dedicated to weaving your words into hope, even when it felt hard to keep believing, has now manifested into reality. It's finally yours, in full validation, with full pay, with all the good. Every single thing, the sacrifice and the beauty, belongs to you because you've been working on this. You earned this.

This *can* be your reality; you can build it. I want the work you're putting into healing to pay off, and *when it does,* I want you to believe you deserve to live in it blissfully.

This may sound strange, but I've met successful people who felt like they'd made it, only to discover they've never been sadder. There are many reasons why this can happen, but I want to focus on when *success becomes your purpose.* Because when you believe *"my purpose is to make it,"* the burden and responsibility of joy is now placed on your goals. Seeing your dreams realized is inspiring and will certainly bring you happiness, but unfortunately, having your dreams come true won't fill you up permanently.

Post-achievement sadness and post-achievement grief are real. The slump that comes after riding those highs is humbling. I know I'm telling you that not even success can be simple; however, I think it's essential to share this because many people are often shocked when these waves of emotions arise. I've struggled with this myself. When you finally figure out how to get what you want, and the chase is over, grief can follow. When people who didn't value you before now think you're a winner because of the shiny things you achieved, grief can follow.

It's not easy knowing the phone is only ringing with invites and dinner dates because of the job you have. It's not easy realizing you were being judged before, and now, after what others believe you've achieved, you belong. You're "in." Yes, there's joy too, but the presence of sadness can be startling amid winning.

I also want to point out that having the mental space and capacity to search for purpose is a privilege, and I want you to lean in to that word. It's a privilege to know how you feel, to be connected to something deeper than what's just on the surface. You're one of the lucky ones, even if it doesn't feel like it, because the alternative is to float through life believing what you have, even if it isn't enough, is all there is.

So, when I ask, "Do you want what you worked for?" I'm asking now that you have it, is it giving you what you believed you'd get by committing to it? Or are you still saying yes because you hoped meeting this goal would get you other meaningful, heart-centered things that can't be bought or earned?

The Arrival Fallacy was coined by Dr. Tal Ben-Shahar, and it discusses what happens when we believe achieving a major goal will lead to lifelong fulfillment.[1] The theory focuses on high achievers—think Olympians, Super Bowl winners, etc.—and how they experience emotional lows after major successes.

I've also seen people who don't fit the "high achiever" or "high success moment" mold experience the post-success slump. I've seen it happen to people post-marriage, post-birth, post–leaving their career to raise the kids (which for many is a massive achievement), post–their kids leaving the nest, post-retirement, post–building their dream business, and post–making their dream number of dollars.

Arrival Fallacy says that when we focus on a goal, we don't always think about what comes afterward. Our lives are dedicated to success and achievement, yet we often have no clear idea of what we want to do once we achieve it. We lose sight of what truly matters to us, and we never question how our actions align with our overall plans for our lives. Wild, I know!

So, do you *still* want it?

This is why choosing something that feels compelling is part of your invitation. **Choice** is one of the Seven C's, so you base your decisions on what you want. **Compelling** is one of the Seven C's, so you make sure your choices matter. **If what you *choose* isn't *compelling*,** because it's just another title behind your name, or another degree, or another thing that you think will fulfill you through validation or spotlight alone, it won't work long term. It will fade.

Our achievements are important. We work, and most of us want to do a good job and be rewarded for it. There's nothing wrong with pursuing big dreams, but that can't be what your life is defined by, or you'll miss the opportunity to have relationships, experiences, and growth from leaning in.

Without understanding your values, you'll live your life trying to answer that big "what's next?" question that we all have when we reach a goal. And you'll find your life becomes defined by trying to answer that question, instead of actually living. Little You has things they want to achieve, but when you're young, that list isn't formed yet, so you shine for the world. Choosing something compelling ensures you satisfy your soul's needs from within.

This is why starting small is so important. We're used to going after massive achievements, so we don't feel the same ping of *"we did it"* energy when we do small things. We shy away from small moments, looking for big tasks to conquer. We keep our plates full because stillness or slowness feels insignificant. However, there can be immense joy in taking a walk, building a magnet house with your kids, grabbing tea with friends, or putting up a bird feeder and watching the birds return each year. These seemingly small things can hopefully be the "why" behind the work you do.

Our ability to be motivated from within is called "intrinsic motivation."[2] It's about harnessing the excitement we feel when we do what we love, rather than doing things out of obligation. It's the difference between "I'm here because I love this work" and "I'm here because they pay me to be here." And with your purpose in mind, this invites you back to the core of who you are and what you're here to experience, beyond your achievements.

While writing this book, I made a promise to myself that I would enjoy the writing process this time. I have "enjoyed" writing my other books, but I put so much pressure on myself to get them *right* that I missed the joy part. My love of writing became my career, and I turned my creativity into strive mode. I still haven't sat down to think about the fact that I've written two books—now three. What a thrill that is! Instead, I asked, "What are the stats?"

Both perspectives are important in business, but if you don't enjoy what you do, as I've said, it will drain you. I'm learning to bring joy into my work, so I don't lose the magic of what I love. I discovered other creative outlets that had nothing to do with my work, allowing me to be creative in other ways.

This is part of intrinsic motivation, which asks us to ask ourselves, What matters beyond success? Beyond status? Beyond validation? By choosing to find joy in the process of turning my idea into something people can read, my purpose extends beyond what the world says about me as an author. My definition of success has been redefined. Everything else comes secondary and thrives from that energy.

> ### Remember for a Moment
>
> When you look back on your life, what moments mattered to you beyond success? What moments became about who you are to the world?

While speaking with folks for this book, I heard so many varied descriptions of what meant the most to them, stories filled with tears and hope.

Deesha is enjoying snow tubing and creating beautiful dinners in her home with friends who spark creativity and build connection. She mentioned,

My husband bought me a sewing machine yesterday. I haven't sewed in fifteen years, but he got it for my birthday. And I kept talking about it and mentioned, "Oh, I want to get a sewing machine, but we're saving for a house and trying to be strict." And with the sewing machine he got me two classes, and it's just like, I'm not going to do anything on New York Fashion Week. But I'm just so excited about making curtains, girl.

Amanda shared:

I just wrapped a group coaching cohort where it was all creative entrepreneurs, and by the end, everyone was like, "I'm sick of my industry. I'm sick of my business. I want to move off the grid." Like, everyone. And what I think is if we had the freedom, we would all be singing in parades, planting flowers, hugging our children, making beautiful things. It's not that we wouldn't be working. It's not that there wouldn't be commerce, but the reason why we choose a lot of these paths is because someone said you had to go work at Goldman Sachs. I know that I'm not in any sort of midlife crisis because the changes I've made have made me so relaxed, and I'm so joyful. I don't have any of the doubt that I used to feel. There's still fears because it's not the most practical path. If I stayed on my other path, I'd be on, like, a *Forbes* list potentially. But there's also this deep clarity and joy that comes from being like, no, what I've chosen is of value.

I talked to a group of friends recently and found myself saying, *"Man, this year was hard. I can't wait for next year, for fresh energy and to start again."* But I realized the only common theme of each year is I'm in it. And if I'm finding it hard each year, I have to look at my expectations, but also what I'm spending my energy on. Because if I'm healthy, have the resources I need to care for myself and my family, and I'm choosing things based on my Seven C's, then something in my belief system about what makes this a "good year" is off. I then jokingly shared with them, *"At some point, I've got to start evaluating if the problem is me."*

This is what I want you to do. There will be parts of the year that rock you. Life is hard, let's not pretend it's not. Death, health issues, job losses, friend breakups, raising teens (need I say more), etc. Of course we feel exhausted sometimes.

But when I looked back on those years that I called hard, I didn't have any of those "hard" things happening. Most of what felt hard was the pressure I put on myself and others, the boundaries I didn't set, and the lack of meaningful things to look forward to daily.

So, I decided to act, and I started small with walking in my neighborhood during sunrise. Not only because I love sunrises but because I wanted to see how they changed each day and throughout the seasons. I'd never felt like I had the time to do this, and I wanted to, so I **committed** to making the time. In the first few weeks, I noticed these walks became about more than just the sunrise. I saw a group of dogs playing in the morning, while people drank their coffee and connected with one another. I recognized people on my walks, and our morning greetings became more than a casual "hi"; we remembered each other every day and smiled. I noticed how the sun changed position each day and how I felt when I got out, even in the rain, when there was no sunrise to view.

Saying yes to a small thing becomes a big thing because you realize what matters to you isn't what you thought. You don't need a big T (trauma) or a significant achievement to witness this perspective shift. Yes, massive change can completely knock you into gratitude, but it doesn't always have to be that way. You can make significant changes, starting with small commitments. You can change your perspective as you figure out your next steps. As always, the choice is yours.

I want you to rediscover your values. How does your job help you love your life? Why are you happy to be married? Why are you happy not to have kids? What are you making space for in the future by saying yes to the hard work now? Ultimately, what are you working so hard for now, and is it worth it?

By asking yourself these questions, you'll establish your Value-Centered Goals, and they'll help you keep going on hard days. You'll remember you're **committed** because you're in this for the long haul. These goals will support the moments that make you look back and say *I'm so glad I did that.* You'll never regret making space and time for the things that make you who you are.

Your Value-Centered Goals, built based on the Seven C's, could look like:

- I want to save ___ [amount of money] to buy a small farm and garden. It will require me to work ___ hours, receive ___ promotions, and make ___ [amount of money], but it's worth it because I'll get to live my dream.

- Having a family is a dream, and the very thought warms my heart. I know there will be sacrifices, I know it won't always be easy, and I know I'll need support. My career-centered goals will help me create space for this dream, allowing me to have the life I desire without the struggle.

- I dream of having more time for volunteer work that I care about. When I was young, I volunteered more often, and it's been hard for me to prioritize because I work a ton. I know that achieving many of my career goals will help me reach the career level I want, but it will also give me access to do what fulfills me. My promotion has come with flexibility, allowing me to leave early on some days, volunteer, and still have time for myself.

- I know I'm sacrificing a lot of what I want to put my kids first, but it's something I know I won't regret. I have lots of things I want to do, but spending time with them when they're small is something I won't be able to re-create. It requires a lot of energy, and I'm exhausted most days, yet it gives me so much meaning. When they go to school or take naps, I find time to dedicate to myself. Creating art on my iPad or writing a few words reminds me I still have dreams I'm making come true that aren't about being a parent.

- I've started a book club. I barely have time for it, and yet it's bringing me so much joy. Having the club holds me accountable because we have scheduled discussions. I've even started using an app that allows me to check out books from a digital library, saving money while still doing what I love.

- I want to travel and have the freedom that being a parent doesn't allow. Instead of building a family, I'm saying yes to relationships, adventure, and freedom.

Value-Centered Goals should align deeply and **confirm** ideas, desires, and dreams. When you're running late to your book club because you're squeezing it in, you'll *still* feel like *there's no other place you'd rather be* since you value it. While volunteering with your kids and schlepping them around in traffic, tiny (or big) attitudes and all, you'll feel like *there's nothing else I'd rather be doing.* When you finally get to plant your first seeds in the garden you saved for, and you watch daily as buds sprout, you'll think to yourself, *I'm so grateful I made space for this.* You will *know* when your goals are aligned with who you are and what you want because even with everything you must sacrifice for them, you'll get **confirmation** from within that you're exactly where you're supposed to be.

I know I'm telling you to find meaning in what you do and also sharing that purpose isn't about what you do, work or otherwise. Both are true; this contradiction is part of the process.

Don't get stuck figuring out why you said yes to things you don't want. Asking yourself challenging questions without a plan to utilize that information to move forward is a trap. You don't need to go back and get justice for lost time unless you plan to use that "why" to help you move forward. Nothing is as stuck as it seems when you're willing to be free.

> ### Come Back to Yourself
>
> Discuss with a friend, your partner, or your therapist/coach about reframing what you've worked for. Lean in to your community. How is what you're doing opening doors for your Value-Centered Goals? How can your life change for the better by helping Little You live their dreams out loud?

in this era,
speak light into your life.
remember,
your truth is your guide.
you know.

9 Rinse + Repeat

We're taught that having peace means experiencing an undisturbed calm, where everything is perfect at work and home, you've *found* yourself, you know who you are, and you're living your purpose. But do you really want to be an ocean with no waves?

In the pursuit of this existence, we keep things as predictable as possible. We find a lane, even if it isn't ours, and we keep it simple—same ol' thing every single day.

The problem? Routines are great until they become a cage. You find yourself locked in the same patterns, sometimes for years, without even noticing how stuck you feel. Part of the reason you don't feel your discomfort is because you're busy, and probably on purpose. It's hard to hear your thoughts, it's hard to connect to Little You, and it's *easy* to ignore your intuition when you don't have time to tune in with yourself.

Your busy life can lead you to mistake being scheduled or booked for satisfaction. You think, *I have so many things to do, so this must be what a full life is.* But "full" and "fulfilled" are two very different things. We busy ourselves to ignore what we don't like about our lives. *I can't think about what isn't working when I'm busy.* The kids grow up, work ends, you retire, you get older, and then you're faced with what you've been running from all along.

Yourself.

Peace doesn't require a life where the ball never drops. Peace is knowing who you are and believing that no matter the circumstances, you can tap into the steadiness within and trust you have what it takes when issues arise. It's knowing that you've built a life that's so beautiful that when the ball drops, you can keep going. No matter what interruptions come your way, they won't sway you.

When we live without variety, one day we wake up searching for ourselves because "the ignoring" we got so good at can no longer be contained. Little You busted out of the cage, and now you're after peace, after knowing, after the wild.

Living a meaningful life will require you to say yes to the unknown. It's begging you to have moments that flow, that are fluid and free. Your younger self had the gift of innocence that helped you say yes to exploring. Your whole world was lit up with thoughts of *I wonder.* You might've thought growing up meant saying goodbye to that part of you, but you're wrong. You might be thinking: *How can I do something different when I've done the same things for five to ten years or more? How can I bring who I was with me, when it feels like that part of me left long ago? The people I know today don't even know that part of me anymore. I don't even know that part of me anymore.*

Before you blame yourself for the rut you're in, remember your brain was wired to choose routine. Even if the patterns, cycles, or rinse-and-repeat rut we're in isn't working for us, we've gotten used to it, so we keep it going. The research I shared in Part I helped us understand how we learn behaviors and how our brains become resistant to changing once we learn to do something one way. Our brains prefer repetition and familiarity to reduce overload and conserve energy overall.

When we do a behavior that we've learned and it goes the way our brains expected, even if it's harmful or something we no longer want to do, dopamine could *still* be released, signaling to our brain *that we should keep doing this*. We're told by our brains to keep doing the rinse-and-repeat cycle even when we want something new, because our brain is like, *"We've got this reward; we should keep going."* This pattern is part of why we feel stuck. This same pattern is why it's challenging to change your eating habits, start reading books, or keep up your daily walks, despite your desire to do so. This is what makes hitting the snooze button easy, even though you dislike being late. This is what makes you choose scrolling endlessly on your phone over taking out your paintbrushes. You're not lazy, you've programmed yourself this way, and it's incredibly hard to change. To change, we must interrupt the behavior.

I hope understanding that we're wired to resist change is a huge relief for you; it was for me. I hope this information helps you stop blaming yourself, because you were *made to learn one way*. It was supposed to be efficient, not problematic. Trying to learn something new is as challenging as it feels for everyone. This is why taking small steps is powerful in creating long-term change, because it slowly shifts the cycle we've been in so that a complete overhaul doesn't jolt us.

This is also why we feel short-term relief when we continue doing the same familiar things; it all helps our brain feel good. I want you to question what you feel, asking yourself, does this *feel good* or *is it just familiar?* We often stay in situations for the sake of having something to do rather than choosing the discomfort of doing nothing until we know what's next; even though the former is a waste of time and energy.

Our brain can mistake our rinse-and-repeat behaviors, unhappy patterns, and repetition for a stable environment, and stability often holds meaning for us. Nothing is rocking this boat, so *everything is good, right?* We think "no waves must mean peace," but check in with your values and ask, is that true?

To change these patterns, we've gotta want it, and beyond wanting it we'll have to be **committed**. We're not just changing our behaviors, we're rewiring how we think. We're **choosing** new ways of rewarding ourselves.

This is one of those healthy **challenges** I was talking about in the Seven C's. When you stretch yourself to do something tough, new, and *challenging,* it builds resilience. Next time you're faced with something challenging, you'll remember that you've accomplished complex tasks and can do them again.

I hope this helps you realize you aren't broken, you aren't a bad person, and you aren't lazy. You're not sitting on that *Imposter syndrome train* or *Who do you think you are train* because you want to be there! Those resolutions you set, those goals you tried to reach, and the things you thought were motivating you were real. The excitement you felt about approaching a new way of living was real. Choosing scrolling on your phone over your creativity, choosing sleeping in over getting up to paint, and choosing to binge-watch a show over making the recipe you planned aren't things you do because you don't care about yourself. It's a pattern that WE have fallen into without noticing what it was doing to us. That first time we said yes to this pattern, we didn't know it would stick for years. We didn't think it would be incredibly hard to break.

The first step? Please forgive yourself.

You didn't intentionally say: *I'm choosing this unhelpful cycle because it's gonna slow down all my plans, dreams, and goals. This is perfect. Everything I think I'm worth won't be possible with this barrier, and I want to make everything more complicated for myself. These unhealthy cycles will last years, and I want to feel like my life is passing me by; I want to feel stuck. I don't care what's best for me; I'm choosing the hard way.*

No one has chosen any harmful experience, partner, friend, or cycle with those words in mind. Quite the opposite: We were hoping for connection, healthy stability, peace, freedom, excitement, joy, and fulfillment. Things don't always turn out the way we expected at first. We can't predict everything that happens in our lives, so please forgive yourself now. If that feels too hard, look your little version of yourself in the face and remember what you want to give them. Allow the frustration to soften when you remember that you still have time to make it easier on them, on you, and build your life. Remember that you're learning the lessons as they come. If a lesson arrives and sticks, that's a blessing. Right?

Next step: Answer this question: What do you want?

We talked about this in the last chapter, and we're here again. If you don't know what you want, then you will for sure stay where you are. Open your mind up to dreaming and carry that new vision with you. What you want right now might not be what you like in the future, and I know it's scary to choose something that might not work; however, staying where you are isn't the answer. Allow fear to spark your memory so you remember how capable you are at succeeding when trying new things.

When Deesha decided to apply for the White House internship, which eventually led to her serving as the White House social secretary under President Barack Obama, she wasn't looking at every single step. Deesha knew she was ready for a change, and that, ultimately, she wanted to contribute to something meaningful. She said, "I was thirty years old, a community college student, and had no political connections. But I knew I wanted to make a difference, so I applied for a White House internship, and it changed my life."

Thirty was never supposed to be our peak, like we've been told via cultural references in magazines and movies. That biological clock concept, beauty and youth standards, and culture in general supported this idea that we now know isn't true for any gender. For many, thirty is the beginning and serves as a launching point. But what if forty is your launch pad? What if you won't hit your stride until your sixties? We'll launch a thousand times if we choose, beyond thirty, beyond forty, and beyond fifty. Many of us believe that we're supposed to have it figured out, but that thinking keeps us from figuring it out. Your only job right now is to answer the question What do you want?

You might be thinking: *What if I genuinely don't know? What if I feel inspired by everything you're saying, what if the research makes sense, what if I'm beginning to believe all of this and yet I still don't even know what I want? What do I do then?*

You start with the first thing you know you want. **Your small wants.** Have you been wanting to buy a new trash can for your bathroom? Have you been meaning to declutter your bathroom cabinets? Have you been meaning to try chili crunch on your eggs? Have you been saying that you want to try making avocado toast at home? Have you been thinking about wearing a monochrome outfit but haven't yet? Have you been wanting to try bangs? Have you been thinking of joining the walking club you read about near your neighborhood? Have you been thinking about writing a post and sharing it on social media?

Start small and lean in. Look up the cost of the new trash can, consider the colors you want in your bathroom, and think about the products you use frequently in your cabinets, as well as the ones you could donate or discard. Research the different chili crunch brands available and their level of spiciness. Think about the avocado toast you've eaten and which bread you liked the best, and add that to your grocery list. Create a Pinterest board so you can see which monochrome outfit excites you the most. Figure out whether you want long bangs or short bangs. Find out when the walking club meets. Start writing two lines for your post and commit to sharing it tomorrow.

By leaning in to your small wants, you give yourself *a win.* Your small wants don't have to be the thing that will change your life, but giving yourself those small wants **will begin to change your life.** Those small wants help you lean in to inspiration and be **creative** in a way you probably haven't in a long time. When you do this, you spark more creativity and more inspiration, and out of nowhere, motivation comes walking through the door. Those small wants become very significant, creating actual changes in who you are, how you perceive your surroundings, what you eat, your style, your activities, and your **community**.

Your small wants reveal that, as scary as change is, it can also be enjoyable. It helps you do things that are more accessible without the overwhelming desire to crush something big. If you gave yourself just one of those small wants I mentioned, you would feel the impact. You'll go to your bathroom and feel exhilarated that you finally picked out the new trash can. You'll curl your bangs each night with joy. You'll go to bed like it will be Christmas morning the next day because that chili crunch is downstairs.

Giving in to those small wants helps you answer the big questions later. Go to a museum. Plant flowers. Make the recipes you saved on your socials. Get out of your routine and back into your life. Then watch how your thoughts begin to change. The inspiration, motivation, and fulfilling life you thought were unreachable will start to be yours, even if only in small ways at first. You'll unlock the parts of you that believed days filled with joy were over for you. They aren't.

Remember, you're saying yes to your **creativity** and **committing** to something that matters. Keep going.

Next question for you: How are you going to get what you want?

We love grandeur. This is why we love watching home renovation shows. We don't see how long it took to update the home. We've seen a couple acquire a house, find contractors, get a design approved, and move into a fully furnished home, all within a TV hour. A massive dream done, including time for commercials! Magic.

We didn't see the bank put the loan on hold to verify their income. We didn't see the new homeowners interviewing numerous contractors before finalizing their decision. We didn't know the budget was far more than they planned, and it wasn't a quick phone call resolution; they had to take equity out on the home they don't even live in. We didn't see how hard they had to work to save up to move. **Committing** to yourself doesn't mean committing to being overwhelmed.

I'm all for doing it big, but big leaps sometimes mean big falls, especially when the dream is new. Please keep that excitement, motivation, and inspiration that's finally got you ready to rebuild your life, but commit to small step after small step.

I'm at the park often with my youngest daughter, and she's learning how to skip every other bar on the monkey bars. This started with her just hanging on the first bar, then she began skimming the sides of the monkey bars. Soon, she got comfortable skipping to the middle of the monkey bars, then jumping down, building confidence that she could handle the fall if she didn't make it across. She was training to trust herself. She's learning to trust the process. She's building confidence by taking small steps. And she's doing it all through play.

So, what are you going to do about it?

You're going to learn to start trusting yourself again by believing you can do new things. You have the power to create change. It isn't easy, and yet that doesn't mean it's impossible. You will trust that the desire you have is enough to take one small step, and if you can take one small step, then you can take another. And you will do this until, when you look back, you can no longer see who you were before. All you can do is look forward to see what's ahead.

You're going to learn to slowly trust the process by not rushing yourself. Each small step is a win. Each time you research is a win. Each time you think about what you want is a win. Each time you build awareness, it's a win. Each lesson you learn is a win. You being in the process of transformation is the win. Your peace is found in this process, even in the midst of the challenges you face.

You're going to learn to slowly build confidence by being brave enough to keep showing up. Some things will be easier to shift than others, and if you try something new in one area of your life, it means you can do it in others too. It's the same you.

You're going to play into purpose by remembering that trying new things, creating new ways of being, and learning to love yourself is a gift. This is not a project, and this is not about pushing through. This is about enjoying the process.

When the new things become old, remember you can reinvent them again. If you find a pattern you've been doing for a long time that still feels good, keep it. Your healing isn't about fixing what's broken; you're not broken. You're not fixing yourself either. You're rediscovering, reshaping, remembering.

Come Back to Yourself

If there's a different way to the grocery store, to pick up your kids, on the way to work, *take it*. It can be nice to challenge the ideas you have about what should be the norm. What do you notice on this new route? Is there a store you didn't know was there? Is there a house you've never seen in the neighborhood you've lived in for years? Is someone refurbishing their home? Notice what happens when you interrupt your routine. Notice how you have new questions, new thoughts, and new ideas.

10 What If I Have to Start Again?

The beauty of looking at your life with compassionate honesty is that you'll see what needs to change without harsh judgment, but the hard part is you'll know things can't continue as they are.

No more pretending your marriage is working anymore; you'll have to figure it out. You can't keep pretending you've got everything handled when you're struggling. And you won't keep pretending you're okay living a life that feels mediocre at best when you want more.

Once you notice those rinse-and-repeat cycles in your life, you can't unsee or unknow what you've learned. What you deemed as *enough* before now has new standards, and those new standards aren't always easy to implement because you might have to start again with yourself and others in unplanned ways that could be uncomfortable.

The people we spend the most time with matter. And we've discussed creating boundaries with friends and family, but what if the most significant drain on your energy is the people in your own household? What if it's your spouse or adult kids? What if it's your in-laws who visit frequently? What if it's your boss, who holds long meetings to gripe over everything?

What if starting again means making big changes that you're not ready or prepared to make because you know they have big consequences? How do you say yes to yourself if the people closest to you feel like the obstacles? What happens if you're not just starting something new, you're starting over? Again?

As soon as you get brave enough to start again, or bet on yourself, you'll begin playing this internal game called *"what's the worst that can happen,"* listing the scary things you believe will come true if you choose yourself.

You'll think the worst that can happen is:

People will think my choices are a mistake.
I won't be able to push through at my job anymore
    (and I might lose it).
I'll lose the only friends I have even though they're
    holding me back.
I'll want more, but won't have any idea how to give it
    to myself.
I might be brave enough to start a new business, but
    what if it fails?
People will talk about me, and I won't be able to
    handle it.

I can only start over if I become rich.
Things might go well, but everything will be different.
Maybe something worse than what I'm imagining
happens, and that's overwhelming.

But I have a bigger and scarier question for you:

What if you keep everything the same, not because it
works, but because you're scared?
What if you live an unfulfilling life because you won't
take charge and do what's best for you?

When fear takes over and you begin to think *the worst,*
remember these lessons we've already talked about:

Little You wasn't afraid to dream big. That means you
have those same fearless qualities within you.

Which Seven C is speaking the loudest? Our fear is
only loud when we give it our full attention, and honestly,
we should listen. But equally, what part of you is ready to
commit, be challenged, or get creative? Give that part of you
the microphone too.

You have no proof that any of these *what ifs* will happen,
and yet I know that doesn't make these worries feel less real.
You have more than enough lived experience to show exactly
why you *should* be afraid. The messages you tell yourself are
important, and what you give your energy to matters. Remember, you feel *stuck* because you held beliefs that weren't
true as facts. You have so much more power than you had
when you were little. Remember that too.

The reason starting again brings up worries is:

1. Part of you is overreacting and getting in the way of doing what's best now to protect yourself from what happened in the past.

AND

2. Part of you knows that staying small is holding some of your relationships together, and your decision to reclaim who you are and start again will end some things.

What if starting again means some things can't remain the same? Does that mean you'd rather not try?

Many of us aren't willing to start again because we know what it'll take, and we don't want to make sacrifices for anything else. I don't know about you, but when I've had to start again, I've felt like I'd already given so much to get where I am, and I don't want to give anything else. I wanted ease more than I wished to change.

We think: *Can what I want happen without me having to do or give anything else?*

I know you want a fresh start without the real-life sacrifices you'll be asked to make, but you won't be walking into this mindlessly. Although your Little You is helping to bring the light back into your life, you, with all the wisdom, experience, and resources, are the one making the decisions. You've made tons of mistakes, and you've found yourself on the other side of all of them. Those lessons will guide you. You're not in this alone.

We've come a long way on this journey. One thing we know to be true is that the part of you that's worried about starting again is the same part of you that decided time and time again it's *easier* to choose comfort over change. It's time to tell that part of you it's wrong. If you're not comfortable with the way things are, you'll have to remind yourself of your why.

Why are you starting again? Why are you reclaiming these parts of yourself? Why is Little You begging you to get on board?

You've focused on the worst things that could happen. Our kind, loving, and scared-to-rock-the-boat selves often go to that side of things first. What about the other side?

What if starting again means:

You find every day is filled with the things that matter to you.
Your relationships grow because you know what you need, and you ask for it.
You take up space and stop playing small out of fear.
You lean in to vulnerability, and you're met with love.
You find your people, and it's easy to be you.

What if the *good feelings* you experience after starting again become "the why" that helps you commit and keep going? What if you grow far beyond what was possible if you'd stayed where you were? The beautiful thing about change is that everyone around you benefits. Whether they leave to find what is for them or walk beside you, your growth empowers everyone to move exactly where they need to be. And beyond them and their choices, because that's not the reason you're choosing transformation, your decision to do what's best for you won't go unnoticed. Our energy is powerful and attracts the vibration we're on. Even though change is scary, it also means things could be better. Instead of living inside of hope, you're living your dreams out loud.

Remember the abandoned parts Little You hid away? They get to live now and be free. Yes, you're carrying your fears, but you're carrying your wisdom too. Your meaningful life is begging you to reconsider what you'll gain over what might be lost. It's begging you to say yes because I promise you it's scarier to keep living for everyone except yourself.

Fear can be medicine that teaches you, reminding you of what you don't want. I know you don't want to wake up one more day with regret, because at least if you wake up with failure, you tried. At least if you wake up with uncertainty about what will happen next, you're not in stagnation.

The fear you feel as you're starting again will melt away, and over time, your body will learn you no longer need a big crisis to get your attention and prompt you to move. Instead, you'll reply to the gentle wake-up call that says, *it's time to shift.* And you'll do it because you know you're worth it.

Remember for a Moment

Was there a time when you were willing to be transformed in any way that was best for you?

What did it feel like to be anchored by your purpose rather than the reactions of those around you?

If you're ready, the next small step is through trust.

You'll have to work on believing you are the kind of person who can be trusted. That you know what's best for you. You'll have to talk about yourself with kindness and not use your past against you. When you decide to make a change and a voice comes up and says, *"It's not gonna work out, why try,"* you'll have to **challenge** this voice by saying, "But I've done it before, can I not do it again?" No one knows everything you've done or experienced like you do, and sometimes we use our past as a weapon to keep us from branching out.

Remember, fear doesn't always mean quit; sometimes it means jump. Fear doesn't always imply staying; sometimes it means go for it. Fear doesn't always mean it isn't for you; sometimes it means you'll have to learn along the way.

How do you know if you trust yourself?

If you're ready to trust, the next small step is to *find your enough.*

When will you be full? When will your life look exactly as you hoped? What kind of house do you need, what type of car will you drive, and how much money will be in the bank? What kind of friends do you have, and what kind of trips do you take? What is enough for you? You're not starting again just for the sake of it; you're starting again with intention.

Get specific. Make a vision board, but also crunch the numbers. You might be surprised at how close you already are to what you want, or how it won't be as complicated as you thought to get there. Don't just dream, get intentional. Research the cost of your dream trips, from flights to the restaurants. What will you wear? What time of year do you want to go? Figure out the tax laws for your new business. Plan the months when you'll rest.

When you define your enough, you'll know exactly what you're working toward. Your purpose will be clear because you're committing to the right amount. Enough is powerful; it's not settling. Enough ensures you're not constantly moving the goalpost. Enough ensures you learn the beauty of stillness. It encourages you to live your life and not make it one big project you're meddling with constantly. It's being well fed. It's being well loved. It's living.

The only way to believe you've done enough is to build your new standards.

Your old life was based on old standards, many of which were created for you. Now that "you know better," as Dr. Maya Angelou said, "do better." And how will you do better? How will you prove to yourself you're choosing you and doing this for you?

You don't need to map this out. You have your Seven C's. You have your values. You know what's a yes and what's a no, or at least you know how to figure that out. Get moving, but pay attention. You'll build your new standards along the way.

When Amanda was faced with the decision of staying in her booming career or choosing something different, she created a new standard of success. When Lia decided to pursue writing, she set a new standard for what it meant to follow her heart. When Deesha chose to be herself with so much societal pressure to do the opposite, she reinforced a standard in her life.

What does it mean to be successful to you now? What does it mean to follow your heart? What skills are you holding on to because they fit your new values? How does your purpose shine in what you've chosen for yourself? There will be a lot of noise and opinions from well-meaning people, telling you what they think you *should* do. Don't get stuck in the cycle of *keeping up*.

Shiny opportunities will present themselves, and even though we both know you have what it takes, if you know it's not for you, practice letting them go. Starting again gives you the flexibility to do things differently than before. Go bravely toward the life you're creating for yourself.

What if this next small decision is the best thing that ever happened to you? What if you look back with gratitude at what you chose for yourself? What if this is the very *yes* you've been waiting for?

Starting again is a gift. It means you still have time to do life exactly as you want.

Come Back to Yourself

Look in the mirror before going to bed or starting your day and say out loud: "I'm ready to start again. I don't have the details, but they will come. Right now, my only work is to get ready." This is an excellent moment to commit to yourself. Feel free to add this reminder to your mirror or a place where you can see it often. Repeat daily until you take that first step.

What a gift it is to remember. You've been introduced to the Seven C's, a beautiful opportunity to acknowledge what matters most in your life, and how you can give it to yourself. No matter what happened in the past, you're always on time. With each small step, you're moving closer to change. It's time to shift. It's a new start. Are you ready?

Blank Slate Energy

MY FRIEND, BY NOW YOU KNOW THE searching was never for what's *out there,* it was within.

The lantern you held to guide you was your inner light.

You had to come back to yourself.

To remember.

And what a sight it is.

You're free.

You carry your wisdom, not knowing what's ahead, but knowing what's possible.

You just left the energy of *what if I have to start again,* but I hope you know, *this is your fresh start.*

This is your comeback.

Because you've *come back home to you.*

It's time to enter your future's past. It's time for blank slate energy.

To your Comeback Era.

11 Pre-Regret

You are living in your future's past.

All the mistakes, lessons, worries, and experiences that Future You will go through haven't even happened yet. Trippy, I know. While your energy is often focused on what you believe you've lost, I invite you to redirect the energy toward what you can have access to right now.

You may not realize it, but this moment is the pre-regret phase. Let me explain.

We recall the precise moment when it felt like we'd reached a point from which it was too hard to recover. We said we would do this job, live in this neighborhood, hang out with these friends, or date this partner for a short period. We've all had a partner who was supposed to be a summer thing, and it went far too long. We've all told ourselves that, in a couple of months, when everything *slows down*, we'll figure everything out. Years later, nothing's slowed down, and we're still here, trying to make a life out of something we knew up front was never supposed to last, whether it's a relationship, career, friendship, or location. It was never supposed to be our whole lives, just a memory.

Now we've reclaimed the parts of us we put away in those moments in the dark. The stories we told ourselves to keep us in ignorant bliss have been recanted and restored. The feelings have been witnessed. And whether you realize it or not, you are no longer just an innocent bystander of your past mishaps. You're standing at the beginning of your future, a future that can be anything you decide.

Pre-regret is the phase you're in **before** you wish you had chosen something different, before you wish you had kept up with your goals. Right now, you're living in the most special time. But when we call it the *present*, your mind gets sucked back into what *was*, right back to the past. It's hard to witness the now and stay grounded in the moment, so your thoughts swim back to what? Your rinse-and-repeat cycles that you deemed monotonous, boring, repressive, and overwhelming. Suddenly, that familiarity of the past looks shiny and new. Suddenly, it wasn't so bad after all. You forget you have a **choice**. Familiarity is a trickster.

Remember when Amanda decided that her successful career wasn't worth the toll it was taking on her body? Remember when she decided to make a change, even when it was **challenging**, even when she was scared? She decided to **choose** something different. The moment she made that *shift,* she moved to a state of pre-regret. Amanda no longer had to *wish she had chosen something different,* because she had decided to do what was best for her future self.

I know you've made mistakes. And let's be honest, those *so-called "mistakes"* are lessons. They feel like land mines because they blow up the lies we held and expose the truth. I know you wished you made different choices and listened to yourself and others. The feeling that if you could go back, you'd undo the pain is real. There are lessons you're learning right now simply because you didn't go with your gut. Life could be different, I hear you.

But you must let yourself off the hook. Realize the time you're in, which feels like it happened yesterday, has passed. You're in a whole new energy. Probably a whole new decade. Yes, you might be working through details. Yes, some of your past choices may now be with you for the rest of your life. I understand. You still get to move forward. Every day you open your eyes, you get to do something new. This is the pre-regret phase. Yesterday's *so-called "mistake"* is not today's mistake. You've brought those memories with you, but they aren't the now. They're from the past.

Living in your future's past, your present, is living in blank slate energy.

You want your future self to look back and say:

I'm so proud I learned to choose me.
Because I prioritized my friendships back then, my life
    is so full.
Thank goodness I got that divorce, because I'm *free*
    today.
If I didn't take that chance ten years ago, I would
    never be here. I'm so thankful for Little Me.

Who you are right now will be the Little You to the Future You. And that's the beauty of living in the pre-regret phase.

We'll have regrets, y'all! That is a part of the human experience. Stuff will happen, and we'll wonder why we did it and how we made it through. And. Tomorrow means blank slate energy. We get to do it all again.

You can have blank slate energy and be accountable.

You can have blank slate energy and be responsible.

You can have blank slate energy and forgive yourself.

You can have blank slate energy and learn the lessons.

You think by holding yourself hostage to your past mistakes, you're ensuring you pay the price and learn, but you're just punishing yourself. Punishment has become a harmful ritual that's keeping you from thriving. It's keeping you from remembering that your responsibility right now is to give yourself a life that fills you up. That's it!

Remember, those *so-called "mistakes"* are behind you.

Little You is not blaming you for learning the hard way. Future You will look back in awe at all you overcame. So why are you mad at yourself? Why are you holding yourself back?

Whenever we want to grow, we're always leaving something behind. Sometimes growth requires more sacrifice than we'd like to admit. To move forward, we dedicate our time, attention, and focus to something new, which means something that had our attention before can no longer receive it. It's time to release the idea that these *so-called "mistakes"* are holding you back.

I know it's hard. Things didn't work out the way you hoped. This feeling sucks, and it doesn't go away until you decide to move forward.

But when you're living in regret, it continues to surge through your body, controlling every move like you're a character in a video game. Sometimes it wakes you up in the middle of the night, like you've had an IV of espresso shot into your veins. You look toward your nightstand to see the time, and you immediately know that you're the kind of awake that isn't going back to sleep anytime soon. It's the kind of awake when what's on your mind is so heavy, so burdensome, that it keeps you from rest. It's as if no time has passed, as if you blinked instead of slept.

When you're in regret, your inner critic is loud.

It will recount all the reasons you should stay where it's comfortable, and fear will slide in too, sharing examples of why your inner critic is right, saying:

"Everyone will judge you."
"There's nothing better than what you have."
"It's far too hard to start again."
"You'll have to do this all alone."

It'll approach all your dreams and desires like a statistician, a doctor, and a researcher, providing you with what it will call "facts." Your job isn't to argue with it. Your job is to hear regret out. Let regret air its grievances. So much of your wisdom lives here. Take the lessons, but leave the fear behind. You get to choose.

Your job is to pursue what you want with faith and assurance that, through your actions, you'll discover your truth, and this is the bravest work you'll do.

Moving from the past, or regret, to your future, or pre-regret, is a gift.

I want you to know that you can lose time. I know we say that *what's for us will never pass us by.* I believe that's true, only if we're still committed to going after it. What's for us can magically fall into our laps, and yet we must still be **committed** to keeping what we've been gifted. If we work for an opportunity, we must show up, so it sticks around. Otherwise, it'll leave, and you'll miss it. And I don't want you to miss it, because we need you living in your gift. The world needs it.

I know that when you look back, you can see moments that, at the time, you didn't realize were special. You were so busy striving, you forgot you were winning. By shifting out of stagnation, **choosing** yourself, and making your life a priority, those special moments aren't missed; you're present, and living them. Blank. Slate. Energy. By taking the chance on yourself today, you won't have to live your life looking through the rearview mirror. You can look right in front of you and witness it yourself.

This is where I want your energy. Not in what you could've or should've done, but in what you don't want to miss now. Remind yourself that everything that's happened has already occurred. There's no more preparation needed for what you've already made it through. You could still be healing from it, and yet, that doesn't have to stop your future. That doesn't stop you now. Thankfully, the things you're here to do can operate without you needing to have it all together.

Believing that there's even a way to *"get our lives together"* is a sham.

You thought that you'd have to understand everything you've done to move forward. But that's fear dressed up in its know-it-all attire, looking like it's helping you be careful when it's holding you back.

How much time have you spent trying to figure it all out?

Healing was never intended to be a block to your future; it's supposed to unlock your gifts. There are times to integrate, times to pause, and times to understand. There will be moments of grief and sadness that shock us out of focus. But that doesn't mean *wait until you've got it all together.*

When we try to live the lie that we can "have it all together," we force our happiness into a confined space. You're telling yourself that nothing can go wrong. You're telling yourself to get it right, to do it perfectly, and to never step out of line. Life isn't designed to be lived that way. Take the chance on yourself.

You're living in your future's past. Anything is possible. You have blank slate energy.

Your life is what you make it, for real, and I hope you choose to trade in your resentment for peace. I hope you know you can live in a zone of pleasure that isn't reliant on perfection. Where something could still be missing, but at least you know you can look for that extra thing *while* enjoying where you are right now. You can begin living right now.

This pre-regret phase serves as a reminder that your purpose is more dependent on your awareness than your actions. I want you to move when you want to move. You'll know you're ready because the answers lie within you, bubbling in every conversation and experience. You'll wake in the morning with more excitement than usual. That dragging feeling of doom won't be at the dinner table with you anymore. The cloud of overwhelming regret hanging over you will give way to clarity. Even when it doesn't turn out the way you hoped, there's no stagnancy unless you choose it because of *so-called "mistakes."* Stagnant energy is where dreams die. That's where we watch time pass and our lives slip away.

For the first time, women are talking publicly about menopause, and I've been learning a lot. The most shocking thing

I discovered is that menopause is just one day. The American College of Obstetricians and Gynecologists states, "Menopause is defined as the permanent cessation of menstruation resulting from the loss of ovarian follicular activity and is recognized to have occurred following twelve consecutive months of amenorrhea." This means menopause is the day that you have gone twelve months without a period. That one day is the sum of one experience, and then the next day, you're in a new phase. A great deal of emphasis has been placed on that one-day term, menopause, without any context of what was happening around it. That's why women are shouting from the rooftops about pre-menopause and peri-menopausal symptoms, because what happens before matters.

This is the same thing we do when a *so-called "mistake"* happens, or we fail, or things don't work out the way we hoped. We put all our focus on that one moment and forget all that came before and all that we can create after.

Remember your intentions. Remember what you learned along the way. Remember.

You didn't choose that partner and think, *This will be a great way to mess up my life.*

You didn't choose that job and think, *I've chosen the perfect thing to stall me for the next five years.*

You didn't become a parent and think, *I'm so excited to lose my sense of self completely.*

Life happened to you; it happens to all of us.

It shocks us, molds us, and changes us.

You can't plan for everything, my love.

You did the best you could. You tried. You left when you were ready, when you felt strong enough. You changed when you were prepared, when you felt wise enough. You grew when it felt safe enough to spread your wings.

You're still doing the best you can right now. If you feel like you're not doing enough, trade your regret for wisdom. We know what to do, right? We get curious. We remember.

> ### *Blank Slate Energy*
>
> How can you stop trying to make something work that is ready to be let go? How can you leave your regrets out of this blank slate energy moment so you can be present now?

Sometimes the past is with you in the present because you dragged it here. We must honor that truth too. But even if you brought it here, you're still in the **now**, not the **then**.

Stop walking around like you're the version of you from before. Love, you are in a state of divine blank slate energy.

And know this, there will be *so-called "mistakes"* again. They are on the way. Before you fall again, as we all will, I hope you remember your future self and your little self are asking your current self to remember where you are. Where are you right now? Look around. All might not appear as it seems.

How are things grander than you imagined?

How are you more powerful than you were before?

I want you to stop being afraid of *so-called "mistakes."*

Why?

Because you've already messed it all up before, this is the beauty of growing older and wiser. You know you've done the craziest things and gotten out of it, thrived after it. Survived. Won!

I mean, let's look at the way we treated our eyebrows from the nineties through the mid- to late-2000s. Messed them all up. Overplucked, overbleached, and overdid everything! We can't hold on to our past the same way we can't get our eyebrows back. But we learned, right? And despite all we did, we're still thriving.

We've referenced "mistakes" as *so-called "mistakes"* many times, but I want to introduce a helpful term I use. The experiences we call "mistakes" have brought us wisdom—we use those experiences to heal, grow, and thrive. They help us make informed decisions, keep us safe, and help us choose joy. We carry them with us everywhere we go.

It reminds me of the spare change we used to have in our car or bag, which we'd use when we needed it—going through the drive-thru, paying an unexpected toll, or offering it to someone in need. I think this is like the *so-called "mistakes"* we carry with us; they're right there when we need them. We're not carrying our mistakes; we're carrying **pocket wisdom.**

Relying on your pocket wisdom is how you build self-trust. That's leaning on your intuition, your gut, your knowing, and your experience. You thought by carrying them around, they were weighing you down, but that's not true. You carry them with you, so you have access to what you need. Anytime you need a reminder, anytime you need a lesson, anytime you want to know how you felt, anytime you need a reference point for what to do, remember your pockets are full of wisdom. There's no reason to fear what's gone wrong because it's filled with lessons for what is still going to arrive. This doesn't make it easier in the moment, I know, but remember you'll make it through.

You are living in your future's past.

The very thing you're working for in the future is counting on you right now. The work happens now, not when everything falls into place. Now.

> **Come Back to Yourself**
>
> What's something Future You needs daily? Please give it to yourself this weekend any way you can. Whether it's chatting with a neighbor, learning a new craft, reading a book, taking a walk, or having water with healing herbs—try to make it as easy and gentle as possible. Think less about materialism and more about the *feelings* you want to carry with you—joy, love, excitement, adventure, peace, and creativity. If you want a garden but live in an apartment, consider planting herbs on your windowsill. If you're going to run a marathon, start with a twenty-minute walk. Start small.

in this era, excuses have expired.
the version of you who was out searching for themselves
is meeting who you're becoming.
it's always been you.

12 What Will You Do with Your Time?

The best part of choosing yourself?

You. Own. Your. Time.

Do you know why people think you're having a crisis when you decide to break out of your mold? It's because you've chosen to live outside of what so many people do: get older, choose sameness, stick with resentment, and stop growing. By choosing yourself, you're deciding to live boldly. Owning your time is a gift like no other.

Now that you own it, what do you want to do with it?

Our family, friendships, romantic partners, work, and hobbies are the key areas of life that we tend to focus on when considering how our time is spent. They say the way we do one thing is the way we do everything, but I've learned that isn't always true when it comes to our personal lives. We could have the healthiest friendships and struggle in romantic ones. We may be the person you can always count on at work, but we struggle to bring that same energy when showing up for ourselves. If you spend significant time with people or in situations that aren't working, your life will show you where your struggles are.

The places you spend most of your time significantly contribute to your sense of purpose in life. As you shift your energy toward creating what you want, I also want you to remember what can take that time away from you.

Remember those numbers I shared earlier in the book regarding your time? Even if you own, give or take, 69 percent of your awake time, it won't feel like you have that much freedom if you're being pulled in directions that don't matter. You might be thinking, *Why didn't she share this earlier in the book? I'm ready to get moving, not deal with relationship stuff.*

I purposely didn't discuss external relationships early on because I wanted you to *choose you* first and focus on what you wanted before we brought others into it. I needed you to remember who you are. I needed you to forgive yourself. I needed you to find kind language toward yourself again. I also needed you to stop making excuses.

You were less likely to do what's best for you when you didn't realize how you were treating yourself. You were less likely to put boundaries in place before you saw what putting those boundaries in place could mean for you. Now that you're motivated to create a life that feels meaningful, I have your full attention, and more importantly, you have your attention. When you were worn out, you were in panic mode, but you remembered how to find calm again. Once calm, I helped you remember how you got to that stuck place. Now that you understand, it's time to put it into practice. It's time to live like you matter.

FRIENDSHIP

In adulthood, our friendships have a direct impact on our sense of **community**, and yet, most of us don't get to spend time with our dear friends as often as we'd like. We hope and work to have the kind of relationships where, no matter how much time has passed, being together feels easy. Spending time with people who enrich your world is life-changing. Knowing in the middle of a hard week that you have dinner planned at a friend's house is life-giving. Having someone remember the hard thing you're going through by sending a text to check on you mid-week is a rich life.

When our relationships don't feel this way, we need to be honest with ourselves. If people in your life are taking up too much time and offering nothing in return, be honest. We've all had those relationships, and as often as we say *"set boundaries,"* we don't often talk about how much time and energy you spend keeping them in place. Everyone isn't interested in ending their relationships, even when they know the person isn't giving them their best. If you're going to maintain relationships that aren't healthy, but that you're not ready to let go of, be honest with yourself about what's happening so you can do what's best for you. This might look like not giving them all your energy if it's not reciprocal, and answering the phone only when you have the energy to be fully present. Redirect your attention to relationships that bring you more.

Do some research about your relationships and be honest with yourself. Are they your friends or acquaintances you know through work? Do your friends provide a safe space for you to be your authentic self? When you are yourself, do they honor who you are? Do you look forward to time with them, or are you not interested in reaching out regularly? Answering these questions helps you be intentional about *who you spend your time with*.

Remember, your job isn't to spend your time trying to change them or attempting to drag them on a healing journey with you. Your job is to accept who they are and allow the friendship to flourish without draining yourself.

Once you shift and stop allowing yourself to be drained in relationships, you'll have space for connections, old and new, from a fresh perspective.

When Deesha chose to be herself despite her powerful position, she prioritized authenticity. She decided to connect based on who she is, not her title, which meant those relationships had a chance to build authentically. Why does this matter? Long after she left her White House role, many of those people remained in her life because they chose Deesha, not her accolades. Be you, always!

Remember, once you've set boundaries and moved through these changes, you're back in your pre-regret phase, and you can make new decisions this time—with blank slate energy. Use your time wisely by leaning into the relationships that fill you up. Don't let past hurts keep you from receiving the beauty of **community** now.

There are so many people you will love who haven't even come into your life yet.

FAMILY

We're born into our families without getting to choose the kind of people our family members will be. You arrive, and your family's systems, beliefs, and ideas become yours unless you choose to release them. Your parents likely adapted some of their rules and beliefs from their parents, and all of you play a role that keeps your family dynamics intact, even if the dynamics are harmful.

Maybe you were the mediator, the person everyone calls when there's an argument or misunderstanding. Are you the quiet one who never ruffles anyone's feathers? Or are you the reliable one who gets things done even if you end up doing it all alone?

When you refuse to continue the same cycles that aren't working for you, things begin to shift in your family dynamics, too. Even though it's hard to break harmful family patterns, when you start to feel better, it **confirms** you're making the right choices for you. Whatever your role was, you won't want validation for playing that part anymore. You'll realize the attention you received was from a place of control, not love. Remember, your family doesn't always put these patterns in place to knowingly hurt you or anyone. We learn and then teach what we've learned. It's up to us to question if it's worth keeping those patterns with us.

As you transform, you may wonder where you fit within your family now. Sometimes families accept your boundaries and champion your healing, and other times they fight your changes because it shakes the foundation of the harmful cycle they live in. This isn't easy work, but remember it's not your job to get everyone to join you. This is about prioritizing yourself and reclaiming your time. Some will come and some won't.

You can love your family and still choose yourself. You can love your family and not be who they think you should be. You can love your family and still maintain healthy boundaries. Letting go of being the person *they needed you to be* will give you massive amounts of your time back. This will be bumpy for a lot of people, but you'll flourish outside of those rough moments.

If you're wondering if a change like this is for you, consider how you feel before the holidays or other family gatherings. If your family lives close by, do you dream of moving away so you can *finally be yourself and escape the drama*? Are you excited to sit around and play card games or watch movies? Are you anticipating the meals you'll eat together and the time you'll spend? Or are you worried for weeks before being with them, feeling the anxiety and anticipation of what will occur, before they even arrive? Are you having arguments in your head to prepare for their arrival, knowing you'll have to defend yourself about something harmless that poses a threat to their belief system? And yes, good times probably exist despite the anxiety, but that's not the question I asked.

> ### *Ask Yourself*
>
> Do you spend your time and energy worrying, fixing, and being responsible for grown people who should be managing themselves? All in the name of being family? Choosing yourself doesn't mean not being there for other people, especially those you love most, but it does mean not betraying yourself.

Listen, this is your life! The codependent, boundary-less relationships and the unhealthy patterns can stop with you. Whoever you thought you had to be to be seen and loved isn't true unless you accept that it is. The time you've spent trying to hold things together, which kept you from having time for yourself, belongs to you now.

Little You didn't get to choose, but you do.

ROMANTIC PARTNERSHIP

When we fall in love with someone, we fall hard. We lose all sense of control, understanding, and we surrender. And then sometimes, we forget to come back to ourselves because part of us believes that this new, beautiful connection we've found is the only thing helping us thrive. When we have a strong sense of who we are, we're more likely to bring that into our romantic relationships. When we struggle to define ourselves, it becomes evident in our relationships as well.

The beautiful thing about partnership is that it should **compel** you to become the best version of yourself, not slow you down or stifle you. We don't want to get lost in our person; we want to find a version of ourselves that we wouldn't have seen had we not met them.

Many people have hoped their romantic partnership would be where they would find their sense of purpose. They hoped that their marriage, their long-term partner, or their decision to build a family together would be *enough*. For some, this is enough, and you feel complete. For most, you've made your relationship a distraction from what is dying to come out of you and into the world.

Losing yourself in falling in love is one of the most beautiful experiences we'll have. Why not let it consume you? It's magical. However, losing your sense of self to your relationship is burdensome, not just for you, but also for your partner. You're now expecting this relationship to give you something that only you can give yourself. This is a recipe for disappointment.

If you're in a romantic partnership, get curious about your expectations around how you've looked to this relationship to fulfill you, and be honest with yourself about all the ways it doesn't. Your partner can't complete you. They can provide you with love, connection, deep understanding, friendship, and so much more, but you're each living your own lives. Your sense of purpose was never meant to come solely from this one person; that's a lot of pressure on everyone involved.

If you're still looking for your romantic partnership, remember yourself in the process. You bring so much joy, beauty, experience, fun, and love to the table. You're not seeking the person who *finally chooses you*, you are finding the person lucky enough to be with you—as you are with them. This is a soul-mirroring experience, a celestial exchange. Your life has meaning when you're single; it doesn't finally begin when you're partnered. It's a new chapter to add to the beautiful life that is already you. And if your friends, family, or others in your life have forgotten that, please build a community that reminds you of your value.

There's nothing wrong with feeling like your "life is complete" once you've found a person to live life with. This is an integral and meaningful part of life to many of us. Keep in mind that your time won't just be spent together—careers, separate groups of friends, families, and responsibilities will pull you in different directions at different times. Knowing what brings you together because of who you are individually is such a beautiful way to honor your time together.

If you don't honor your individuality, you might blame your partner for how your life doesn't feel like yours. Your relationship will change how much time you have for everything in your life, yes, but don't forget about Little You.

Your partner may need you, but you need you too.

CAREER

Now that you're ready to spend your time with intention, let's tackle your career, which can be challenging. Career is the most focused-on area associated with our purpose. We have bills to pay, so the thought of cutting back on work to prioritize non–money-making tasks can be overwhelming.

Part of our career goal is to feel connected to what we're doing, rather than focusing on recognition, pay, or other benefits associated with our work. I want to be very clear here, doing work for free does not mean you're living in your purpose. Receiving less than you deserve doesn't signify purpose. Being humble doesn't mean devaluing yourself.

Instead, I hope that when you spend your time working, it feels like a valuable place to put your energy.

For example, my mission is to help people feel like attaining what they want in life is easier after they've spent time with me. I aim to provide people with helpful language for their relationships and conversations. I want people to feel empowered.

When I said yes to my purpose through healing and writing, I also said yes to much more than the business side of things. I said yes to sitting with people in their darkest moments. I said yes to helping people feel witnessed, sometimes for the first time. I said yes to watching people's lives transform. Saying yes to this part of my purpose has changed me in ways I would've never experienced had I not followed this journey. We get both the good and the complex parts in life.

We've all held jobs because we needed health insurance. I've had jobs that helped pay for college and other bills. Everything won't mean something in the moment. But all the jobs of my past that I thought were pointless have been something I've leaned on while working in the job I'm fully aligned with today. It's all given me pocket wisdom, or at least I try to use it all for good. Perspective is everything.

I say all of this because some of us will work in careers that we don't feel a connection to. Then some of us will do something that others deem incredibly small, yet we will feel a sense of pride in everyday life. I recall watching a video on social media about a man who worked for the city of New York's transportation system, the MTA, specifically cleaning the trains. And when I say cleaning, I mean mopping, bleaching, wiping down seats, getting rid of trash, everything. We've already talked about trains earlier, but if you've never ridden on an NYC train, know that they are filthy. I fully bow down to the people who clean them because they are doing BIG work. When he talked about his job, he shared how he had a tiny window, something like fifteen minutes or less, to clean the trains before they had to be off again to start their route.

However, he took great pride in his work. He knew his role helped keep the entire system running, which meant a great deal to the millions of people commuting. He loved knowing that people on the train would feel comfortable, safe, and clean. He knew every part of the process and spoke with respect about every person's job who worked with him. And why wouldn't he? It is a dignified job. It does matter. It's genuinely only how we choose to look at things that impacts how we feel about what we do. Yes, he may have other dreams and desires for his life, but he's found a way to find meaning in what he does. Finding a positive perspective in what we do is something I think would help free all of us.

Your career will take up most of your time and attention. Finding meaning in what we do, even if it **challenges** the standards and beliefs the world has about us, is hard but beautiful work. If what you **choose** to do in the world brings you joy and matters to you, that's enough. Don't be afraid to innovate and bring your **creativity** into what you do.

Lia had spent a great deal of her career on the opposite side of the table from her clients, holding a safe space for their stories as a therapist. She **committed** to bringing her creativity into her work when she started writing vulnerably about her own life. The transition from being a space holder to doing what fills her, and allowing others to hold space for her, is such a beautiful way to own who she is.

Your career is meaningful, but it's not the only thing that matters. Please avoid making your career the thing you believe will change everything else. Little You has always known this wasn't true.

Your awake time is about more than working. Your gifts are about more than working. Everything you're good at doesn't have to become a business. Not everything you create is meant to be sold. But when it's your job, your work, your career, find a way to bring your love to it. You may leave this career eventually, and if you don't like your job, I hope you find something you love. But until you do, by finding a way to bring your love to what you don't like, you'll be choosing to connect with what matters, not just the negativity. Again, it's the *both and*.

Your boss could be the worst, your coworkers may not get

you, and you could know it's time to leave. Receive what's in it for you, give the gifts you bring to the table, and then go. If you can't go right away, plan. And if planning feels too much, dream. Start small where you are.

HOBBIES

Are there museums you've always wanted to visit in your hometown? Is there a restaurant you drive by that you've been meaning to go into, but the day hasn't come? What do you love that needs no explanation, because it makes you feel alive? Have you always wanted to carry around your camera and take pictures of your favorite trees at the park? Do you want to try to re-create your favorite artists' paintings? What fills you? Hobbies are one of the most important things you'll do as an adult because they fill your **creative** cup, inspire you, and help you shine brighter in every area of your life.

But there's one thing that often comes to mind when we think about hobbies that block us. Money. Most of us barely feel like we have enough to be adults, let alone set aside money for things we do for enjoyment. I beg you to give what I'm about to say a try because it's free.

When I started thinking about hobbies for myself, I didn't realize how much I thrived on alone time until I grew up, because my home life as a child didn't give me the space to explore it. Having a sister, sharing a room, and living in very close quarters meant I'd almost certainly have someone knocking at the bathroom door and screaming at me to *hurry up* if I took too long. That was just the way it was, and I loved it, to be honest.

However, I learned something new about myself when I got my own space. Being alone, in silence and stillness, recharged me. And trust me, I love getting together with people. I thrive on having strong relationships. But when I spend moments alone, I learn about myself in a way I couldn't otherwise.

It costs you nothing to get to know yourself alone, and you'll be surprised by what you learn about the ways you like to spend your time. You won't have to be the trip planner for the whole family; you'll get to be you. You won't have to compromise on what your friends want; you'll get to be you. On the surface, you might think you like doing the things you always plan for others in your life, but what happens when you only have yourself? Is that still how you want to spend your time?

When I ask people what lights them up, it's rarely the big things. It's almost *always* the small things. *I'm setting some time aside to paint this weekend. I finally planted tulips in time to see them bloom this spring. I'm hiking that trail I've driven by so many times. I'm finishing the last book in a series I started a year ago.* Those are things that mean so much because they represent what <u>you</u> like. It's not easy making space for the small things, but it's rewarding.

Experiencing the sunrise on a solo walk can be meaningful. It might also be something you invite people you love to do with you too. Going to a movie you've been dying to see, even if no one else can make it, might be something you enjoy. Learning to dance salsa at a free salsa night near your house might be the thing you need for a night of fun.

As important as community is, so is learning to love yourself and be with yourself when you're alone. As we get older, things change drastically. One day, your kids, if you have them, will leave the house. People move. Shifts happen in our relationships. And the one thing that will remain is the relationship we have with ourselves. Make it one you look forward to. Make it one that enriches everything else you do in your life. Make it one that mirrors how much you are loved, not only by yourself, but also by others.

Remember, Little You always enjoyed your company. Turn toward the opportunity to love on you.

The whole you.

Come Back to Yourself

Ask yourself which one of these areas connected with you the most: friendships, family, romantic relationships, careers, or hobbies. Then answer this question out loud when you are alone: What have you been afraid to admit that you know is true?

in this era,
everything you miss,
was never for you.
let it leave.
you deserve to let go with ease.
you deserve to start again with ease.

13 The Whole You

We are gatherers.

Gatherers of evidence, information, and wisdom. When we don't understand or believe something's possible because we've come across it for the first time, we reach into our metaphorical Rolodex for information from our past that helps us understand what's being explained or what we're witnessing.

Even though in the present day you *know* what you're capable of, you question whether you're *really* capable. Can you get through this? Can you keep coming back to yourself? With no clear path ahead?

In moments like these, it's helpful to rely on what I call *my mentors in my mind,* a gift of pocket wisdom that always stays with me. When I needed a mentor, I knew it might take time to find someone who was a good fit for me and vice versa. Mentorship isn't just about receiving; it's a reciprocal relationship that's built over time. To give myself what I needed while I waited for real-life mentorship to form, I started relying on my mentors in my mind's life experiences.

These mentors are a council that I don't know personally, but I still call on them to remind me of a few things:

1. **I'm not alone in my experience.** I'm not the first person to go through this, and I'm not experiencing this because I'm *broken*.

2. **They made it through, and I will too.** You don't have to do exactly what they did, but having an example is helpful for getting unstuck.

3. **They give me language.** When you're choosing something new, you might not have the words to express what you need, because you don't know what could help. But the moment you see someone else going through a similar journey and they explain what they were feeling or experiencing, it's a reminder of what can be helpful to you. You will feel less alone and be more likely to advocate for yourself.

For example, imagine you're having a difficult moment with a friend or at work where you're questioning your worth, something I've done before. This is a moment when you could call on your mentor in your mind. For me, I'd call on Dr. Maya Angelou, one of my fondest mentors in my mind, and I'd think about these words she's written: "My great hope is to laugh as much as I cry; to get my work done and try to love somebody and have the courage to accept the love in return." These words remind me that, in equal measure, life is about the ups and downs. It reminds me that living is a vulnerable experience and to accept love as much as I'm willing to give it. That being deserving of love is my birthright, as it is for all of us. These words always remind me that the feelings I'm experiencing, whether they're hard or abundant, all bring me back to love. And that reminds me to keep going no matter what.

We don't always have people around us who understand what we're going through. Maybe none of your friends have a family of their own yet. Perhaps you're the first person in your family to start a business. Maybe you have no preparation for what you've chosen, but you know it needs to be done. **Community** is one of the most essential things in my life, but I also know that we can't make the people around us fit our goals, our lives, or our dreams. You could be fully supported and *still* have no tangible help with what you're trying to achieve, and that's why I started turning to these mentors in my head. (It's also why I decided to add other stories in this book.)

When you finally find the courage to start taking action in your life and things don't shift as quickly as you hoped, or you don't know where to begin, or you don't have help, or no one wants to take the time, you might start to question the entire process. *Is this even worth it?* This is especially true if you don't have anyone in your life who can remind you that this part that feels a bit lonely is not a personal attack, it's part of the process of expansion. This is part of the change. This is part of deciding to do things differently. This is part of breaking away from doing the same things over and over. Blank slate energy also means not having a blueprint, which is challenging but also exciting. You become in control of your destiny.

A friend sent me this quote, and I've searched endlessly to try and find the author: "I am full of restless energy. The wind outside howls, as if it, too, is unsatisfied. I have so many ideas, but how do I shape them? I want to be brilliant, unforgettable, but what if I am merely ordinary?" The writer of this quote brilliantly shares what so many of us feel deep down.

What if my grand plans aren't as special as I thought they were? What if I'm not as talented as I thought I was? What if this blank slate energy doesn't suit me? What if I'm not cut out to figure it out on my own? I've never done anything on my own.

We've all had these thoughts.

You have to decide that the feeling within you, which reminds you that you're special and that what you want to do matters, is more important than every other thought, even if you have no proof. Especially when we have no evidence, and that's when having the mentors pays off.

You may find, when talking with mentors in your mind or in real life, that the significant disconnect between where you are and where you want to be lies between *who you believe yourself to be and who you actually are.* Are you able to see the greatness that others see in you? Do you recognize the capabilities within you that others admire? Are you willing to acknowledge the growth that's already taken place and how it's no small feat that you've made it to where you are?

You aren't some minor afterthought. No matter where you grew up. No matter who your parents were. No matter what anyone told you. You are valuable. You are precious. You are unique. By connecting with the people you look up to, even if you don't know them in real life, you're building a positive internal **community** within. When you're in tough times, you can recite their positive words to yourself, and it builds a reserve of goodness within, helping you lean on someone whose path you trust outside of your own. Their lessons and mistakes are more **pocket wisdom** you can add to your stash.

Sometimes, thinking about the mentors in our minds and retracing their steps and stories can remind us that everyone has come from somewhere. You see them in all their glory today, but you don't see everything they've walked through to be who they are. You don't know what they're still struggling with, the regrets and pains they held and had to learn to move past. Life wasn't always as shiny as you paint their story to be. Sometimes it was **challenging**, and they had to find **creative** ways to make it through. Remove them from the pedestal on which you placed them, and remember that they didn't always have the answers. It took time. It took patience. Give yourself some of that same grace. You're not any different.

Take One Small Step: I invite you to write a short letter to yourself pretending to be one of the mentors in your mind, and imagine their responses. What do you think they'd tell you to do? What new adventure would they encourage you to try? When would they smile at your choices, and when would they encourage you to go deeper? What would you do after receiving their loving advice? Allow yourself to dream. Allow yourself to think it through, even if the letter is only a few sentences or a voicenote. When restless energy arises, remember that you don't have to have all the answers.

Take Another Small Step: I invite you to embrace patience with the energy of knowing that what feels like a *slow* *season* or restlessness could also be you creating something new. There's so much you've made come true in your life that you haven't even stopped to enjoy. This is your season to finally not be "on to the next." To not slide past your progress. To stop moving on as if you didn't just have a whole breakthrough. Acknowledge that yes, time is passing, and that's an invitation to savor it. Perhaps this is the moment for you to reflect and soak in everything you've created for yourself. Have you allowed yourself to take it all in?

Spending time with the mentors in your mind is also helpful when you're not ready to share with the people in your life what you've decided to go after. I believe in protecting our dreams in their infant stage. In the beginning, they are delicate. They need care, nourishment, and someone who believes in them. Dreams need excitement and delusion to grow. In the dreaming process, you don't need to hear how hard it will be; not yet. You don't need to hear how no one like you has ever done this. You need imagination and magic.

The moment when you need to follow the steps, and to cross the t's and dot the i's, is coming. But you can't put the cart before the horse, if you know what I mean. Everything starts from within first. Everything starts with your belief. Everything begins when you dream.

Think about the mentors in your mind and the things that inspire you. I know they weren't all grand things. Some of what enamors you about the mentors in your mind are accessible things that you can allow to inspire you.

Being the whole you is why we say yes to this work in the first place. When we move into our purpose, our entire being comes alive. I've seen so many people do therapy for years, take tons of courses, read almost every self-help book, go on retreats, journal every day, and do all the things we consider healing. However, healing became a trap because they were *doing the work*, without allowing it to lead them toward building a life.

At some point, liberation must be the choice. Using what you've encountered as the guidance you can lean on as you move through life is the work. Making peace with your past isn't about living in absolute harmony; it's so you can witness how you've been fearless in the face of so much adversity and still thrived. Use that resilience to your advantage. You've had hard times, *and* they've helped shape you into a limitless person. I hope you hold this near to you.

I know some of us have been in therapy for years, reading self-help books for even longer, and trying to put it all into practice. We follow the big wellness influencers on social media and we've drunk the green juice. But we don't see it working in our lives. It's not working because we're not necessarily looking to add more things to our to-do list that look wellness-y. We're committing to making changes that shift our lives. This is the work.

We live in the *and* space, between the past *and* the future. Between who we were *and* who we're becoming. Between who the world thinks we are *and* who we really are.

You might struggle with living in this space because our world has asked you to pick a team, pick a partner, pick a place, and make it permanent. Living in the space of *and* gives us time to integrate. If you've recently separated *and* are ready to date, you can tell yourself, *"I trust you,"* and start putting yourself out there. If you've only been at that job for six months *and* you know you won't be able to stay the whole year, you can say to yourself, *"I trust you,"* and create a plan for what comes next. If you want to move to a new location *and* are unsure whether you prefer the beach or the mountains, consider visiting *both*. You can trust yourself and trust that when you decide, it's the truth. It may not be the truth next year, but right now it's the truth. This is the beauty of the pre-regret phase.

Living in the in-between is not the same as living in limbo. Limbo makes it hard to have any movement, in any direction, because you're stuck. You don't know which way you want to go or if you want to *go* at all. The in-between space is not stagnation; it's a place of expansion. Perhaps your career feels uncertain, while your family life is going well. Maybe you're learning to forgive yourself for your past, and you know exactly what you want next year, the future, to feel like.

Take the pressure off yourself about what comes next or what you need to do now. What if this is what flow looks like for you, a buffet of trying what works and releasing what doesn't with ease? "What if" allows you to be all the things you want at once, without having to pick a lane, because you've decided. You.

Britt's story is one of my favorites about owning *and*. It takes a lot of courage to balance being a powerhouse speaker, author, and expert in a very academic field *with* being a fierce member of the circus. But here she is, living in the *and*, despite what people may think or want for her.

And is where play comes to live and sets the stage for purpose to grow. Our creativity and imagination thrive when we begin to say, okay, maybe I can live in the space of *and*, in the in-between, and say yes until I'm ready for something different. This is what *making space* is. This is what holding space for yourself looks like. What if your capacity for what's possible grew bigger than you ever imagined? What if you allowed what's meant for you to unfold without knowing where it will lead?

What does *and* look like in practice? You might be a teacher for a fourth-grade class during the day, but in the evening, you lead a run club, and on the weekends, you do short road trips to connect with your travel bug. You're a teacher who likes to help children, *and* you're a runner *and* you're a traveler. *And.* You're all those things we listed *and* so much more. You're not just defined by what you do either. You could be a spiritual being *and* a seeker *and* someone who feels led to experience different cultures for growth. You get to be many things *and* all of them can be true.

In the simplest of terms? *And* allows us to exercise **choice**.

"If it's meant for me, I will walk toward it" is a prayer or mantra I encourage you to adopt. It's a reminder that if you say yes, as long as you are willing to meet fate where it lies, fate will show up for you too *if it's meant to*. So often, we take redirections and failures as evidence that we don't have what it takes, when in fact, they are bringing us to *what is meant for us.* There are people and situations that we worked hard to keep, but that were meant to leave. They were only meant to be a season, an era. But we kept them because we became collectors, gathering everyone and everything around us. Our lives become crowded, and we struggle to find ourselves.

It's time to declutter, my friend, so that you don't have to work hard to locate yourself.

If we compare this decluttering to actual spring cleaning, you usually decide to get rid of things because you need space in your closet. However, in an attempt to make space, we sometimes overdo it with our giveaways. When we're finished sorting our piles, we realize there's almost nothing left, which almost always prompts us to go out and get *more*. Getting rid of the things we need or love is pointless because we'll end up replacing them anyway. The truth? Maybe you had enough space, but things weren't arranged in the best way. Some things needed to go; perhaps they no longer fit, you never really liked them, or you had other options that you used more frequently. It's a process, but when you're done, you feel fresh, renewed, and a sense of release.

In the same way, it's time to organize the keep pile, the go pile, and the recycle pile in your life. It's time for everything—your memories, your lessons, your worries, and even the places you struggle to forgive yourself—to have a place, so you know there's enough room for you to exist. Unfortunately, we'll experience things we never wanted to happen, but life brought them anyway. When we've moved through it, we can decide to let those things go. And sometimes, even though we didn't want it, we may choose to hold on because of the wisdom it brought us.

Do you believe in coincidences? Or do you think it's all happening for your good?

Whichever side of the coin you choose, I hope you know you can still land exactly where you're meant to. When you give yourself permission to be whole, you're unstoppable. You build a relentless trust in yourself that allows you to hear your *authentic voice*. If you've struggled to know the difference between your intuition and fear, know that you're not alone, and it takes practice to understand what's helpful and what's not.

You'll know your inner voice is helpful if it sounds like:

I'm scared, but I'm gonna try anyway.
Am I taking this next step because I want to, or because of what others will think about me?
I don't have the time to take anything else on; I want this, but it's not the right moment.

You'll know your inner voice is a hindrance if it sounds like:

Maybe starting feels hard because I don't have what it takes.
Going for that job will end in disappointment; don't do it.
You tried to make it work, and look how this ended? Never let your guard down again.

The helpful inner voice does carry fear, but it's less judgmental. It's motivating while still asking you to get curious about why you're choosing what you do. The harmful inner voice says similar things to the helpful inner voice, but with the addition of negativity, self-loathing, and shutting you down. Learning which inner voice to give your power to will change the way you talk to and about yourself.

Being whole isn't about being perfect; it's about being comfortable not having it all figured out. Living in the in-between may look like you have everything figured out because people see you doing things they're too afraid to do for themselves. They'll say to you and to themselves: *You're different. You're smarter. You've got more to offer.* They'll compare themselves to you the same way you compared yourself to others. We're never more alone than when we're comparing ourselves to someone else.

But you'll know the truth because you did the work. You're just like them and all the other people you once believed cracked some life code that you weren't in on. The only difference between them and you is that you learned to trust yourself enough to take a risk and fall. You're willing to fall because you know you'll catch yourself. And if you don't catch yourself, you know you have a community willing to support you through it.

People assume that a **community** is a vast group. For some, there will be a good-sized group of people—maybe four or five—who you can rely on to be there no matter what you bring their way. But for most, it may be a couple of people, literally one or two, who remind you of who you are when you've fallen so hard that you've entirely forgotten. They'll be willing to pick you up and keep you from returning to your past cycles of stagnation, pretending, or ignoring you.

There will also be your greater community, like associates, friends, and people you trust in your life. They might not be your closest friends, but they are still people you can call on to ask for help when you need support in hard times. Maybe they direct you to the hiring recruiter they know well, or they share a story about a time they struggled to provide the boost you need to keep going.

All the Little Yous that live within you are another community that matters too. Six-year-old you who performed in front of the whole school and was so proud. Ten-year-old you who first tried to protect you from the "friends" who were talking behind your back. Thirteen-year-old you, who didn't know whom to turn to when they started feeling like they weren't enough, to themselves or anyone else, so they chose perfection as protection. Sixteen-year-old you who thought they were surely in this life alone, and would have to learn to survive it or sink while trying. Twenty-year-old you, who believed the only way to make it through was to get it done alone because no one ever does what they say they will do. Twenty-eight-year-old you who couldn't believe how close they were to thirty and how they hadn't accomplished enough, completely ignoring all the work that was put in. Thirty-three-year-old you who refused to give up on love. A thirty-six-year-old you who was becoming worn out from life, and began to feel like *this is just the way it always will be*. You're not only turning to Little You for times you succeeded, you're also looking back to remember how you prevailed.

Every single version of Little You is a member of your internal community, right along with those mentors in your mind. They show up with the right scene from your past or wisdom from previous experiences to remind you of who you are. When you're willing to love yourself, connect with yourself, hold yourself, forgive yourself, rest with yourself, create with yourself, you're bringing the whole you alive.

I know it's been a long journey, but I hope you still have a long journey ahead of you. The longest, to be honest. I know it hasn't always been easy, and I hope that somehow, things are made easier for you. I know you've often had to figure it out alone, and I hope those days of suffering in solitude are long behind you.

You have gifts inside you waiting to bloom, and that's a miracle. So many of us leave this earth feeling alone because our dreams are buried deep within us. You can do it differently.

A life entirely free, being exactly who you are.

Come Back to Yourself

You're not just here to practice healing, you're here to live. So let's create the language, the mantra, that you'll carry with you. Choose words, phrases, or pictures. Write your own or let the mentors in your mind supply the language with their quotes. Let this be your ongoing dialogue that changes based on what you need. Spend five minutes a week adding to or editing this language. Keep it close where you can recite it whenever you need.

14 A Life Without Pretending

The seat is warm and comfy.

We've been riding the train for years, moving in the wrong direction. We've passed our familiar stops: Imposter Station, Who Do You Think You Are Street, and It'll Never Happen for You Terminal. We've sat in that warm seat and let ourselves feel limited because it felt like the only choice. However, we now know it isn't. Just because we've passed through these stations doesn't mean we've arrived at our ultimate destination. We can get up and choose a different route. We can say yes to something else.

When you get on the next train, it won't feel *right* at first, but trust me, you'll feel proud. Despite how hard it was to get off that comfortable, warm seat and keep riding to those same familiar stops. You changed the way you talk to yourself and implemented new language that nourishes your soul instead of draining it. You've decided it's time to be on your own side.

That internal PA system will still say some of the old familiar things that kept you stuck in the past. *Are you sure you want to do this? Do you have what it takes? Are you willing to go this alone?* Those questions will give you pause, and you'll wonder if those questions come as a warning, perhaps to save you from falling flat on your face. That new cold seat will feel even colder in the face of uncertainty. Although it's cold and new, you'll know that for once, you're honoring your future. You're not pretending, you're free. And you're moving ahead.

When you decide to change your environment, you gain confidence. Your energy gives "I'm the one" vibes, and it brings people and experiences into your life that felt impossible before. Remember when we discussed that your actions will **confirm** that the changes you're making are the right ones? This is it, my friend.

Some of us don't know why we feel we're here for something bigger, but we know it was a feeling we were born with. This might scare the people around you, even if they love you, but remember their reaction has nothing to do with you; they're scared because they haven't said yes to themselves yet. When you say yes to yourself, you can't help but root wildly for the person reaching for themselves too. You become a light for them when they can't see the way. When you're around someone who hasn't chosen themselves, your yes to yourself becomes a reflection of their no to themselves. They'll start believing that you carry a level of confidence that keeps you on higher ground than everyone else, and they'll use this against you to protect themselves. It's all projection but it works well to bring us down when we don't yet know who we are. Their negativity can confuse you, causing conflict with your truth. When you share your wins, they'll feel personally attacked. When you dream, they'll feel personally attacked. So, sitting on that cold, new seat and going in a new direction is more than just brave. It's a test. People will be triggered by your decision to go for it.

Your body knows what's happening. That's why when you've gone to dinner with people you don't feel safe with, you feel the response in your body, you feel yourself pushing through. We've all spent time praying that certain people don't show up to events, so we feel safe and have a good time. You've accepted invitations and said yes to meetings that made you feel like you wanted to jump out of your skin and run. Yes, adulting means sometimes doing things that don't feel comfortable. However, sometimes we've said yes to things that we physically know aren't right for us.

Why do we do this? Sometimes, these uncomfortable people are all we have. We tell ourselves they're the only person who can do this job. Or they're in our family. Or they're a person we've known a long time who isn't gonna change. Or, and I must name this one, we knew from the beginning they weren't good for us, but we ignored it and pretended all would be well *eventually*.

Ultimately, we often *do* this because we're afraid to be alone. We don't realize that saying yes to people like this means we're more alone than ever.

We pretend everything is fine when it isn't, hoping we'll feel what it's like to belong. In our communities, with our people, and with our lovers. There's nothing more complicated than feeling like you're an outsider in your own family. Or constantly being told in subtle or direct ways that you're too much, even though you're only asking for the minimum.

When this happens to us after we've finally gotten brave enough and listened to our little selves, it sends a clear message. Move on. Before changing trains, you would've put on the show, but you *believe* yourself now in a way you didn't before.

These uncomfortable moments you would've tried to ignore before are now unbearable. Being with them feels like sitting too close to a cactus. It's not touching you, but with the wrong move, you know you'll get pricked. And we've had enough of sitting close to something that could harm us in the name of love for them. Hoping they would change kept us stuck. But now we're learning to love ourselves enough to stop allowing their projections to be our responsibility. We're no longer carrying their issues as our own.

The people who've committed to not changing will not decide to get it together once you choose yourself. They usually decide to jump ship. Although some leave silently, others walk away with the ferociousness of a three-year-old who doesn't want to go to bed, and it makes what already felt like going after the impossible even harder to bear.

I know you didn't sign up for this. You probably thought, *I will be myself, I will live in my truth, and everything will align.* Things are aligning, but as I said in my first book, *The Sugar Jar*, everyone will not be coming with you. You might be riding alone on the new train for a while because you have boundaries now, and some people only said yes to relationships with you because they knew you didn't have any. Your lack of boundaries was a bonus when they realized a person without boundaries gives more than they have, does things they don't want to, and you can usually take from them with little effort or consequences.

A life without pretending means a life filled with a new perspective on your relationships, friends, and connections. It means that you aren't pretending everything is good when it isn't. It means you're honoring when the answer is no. It means that people won't have as much access to you as they used to. In short, your boundaries will naturally change the nature of everything you do.

Your boundaries will naturally change the way you show up with you too. Be gentle with yourself and know that pretending was something you did out of love, but remind yourself that it isn't a tool you need to lean on anymore. It doesn't mean you won't care what anyone thinks. It doesn't mean that you won't get hurt when people disappoint you. It just means you won't allow those experiences to keep you from doing what you know you're here to do.

Not everyone will be cheering for you. Everyone won't be excited about these new changes. The fears you had about people deciding to walk away from you will be realized. The beliefs you had about no longer belonging in certain groups will prove accurate. It won't be because something is wrong with you. It'll be because you *never* fit, and now you're honoring that truth by living the way you want to.

When you say yes to the life you want, you won't have time for people who say no to it. You'll naturally begin to separate, sometimes without even trying. Growing apart is a real thing, and it's a painful experience. It's why choosing carefully who you have around you is everything, because you will unintentionally limit your thoughts, your beliefs, and your life to what you think will be acceptable to the surrounding people. Pretending.

On this new train, you'll be willing to walk away from

ultimatums that challenge your values. You won't stay with a partner who doesn't respect you, merely hoping for the best. You won't keep "friends" who are jealous of the wins you're making.

You won't be afraid to burn bridges that need to be lit when you acknowledge that some of the people in your life are willing to watch your whole world crash if it means they could remain comfortable. It's time to let them go. The hardest part is finding the courage to do it.

I know this sounds harsh, but it's temporary. The separations, endings, and boundary-led changes won't last forever. In the moment, it will be some of the most challenging work you've ever done. But on the other side of it, you will be free of many of the people, places, and experiences that were contributing to your limited feelings.

Although the initial changes are challenging, you need them. Say yes to them. Welcome them with open arms, knowing your self-worth is more than who they want you to pretend to be. You deserve to show up.

A life without pretending requires people in it who don't expect you to perform for them. It doesn't mean every single relationship will end, but transformations will take place and things won't be the same as they used to be; you'll feel it. You may have to build a new village, and I know this is challenging, especially as we get older. However, not everyone is interested in coming with you as you grow.

This is good news. I know this doesn't sound like a positive, but it is. Who wants to be around people who are holding them back? Who wants to be limited just because someone doesn't think what you believe is possible?

The truth is you're magnificent. Your tone of genius is

only held back by your self-imposed limitations. Not everyone has had a crew of folks rooting for them along the way. For those who have, it still hasn't always felt safe to step out into life on their own and *really* do this. No mask.

But you'll notice a difference in what you say to yourself because there's nothing more for you to prove to them or yourself.

A life without pretending will invite you into the conversations you were able to avoid when you just went with the flow, even when you knew it wasn't a fit. It may not feel like a shift is possible from deciding to get off that train that brings you to the same cycle, but it is.

When you say yes and decide to move forward, that PA system will blast the affirmations that now exist within you.

> *You've done it before, of course you can do it again.*
> *You've already done the most challenging part by taking*
> *the first step; keep going.*
> *They don't believe it's possible for you because they don't*
> *think it's possible for them. Don't let them stop you.*

Many of us don't pursue what we want because we often envision doing it with someone by our side, whether a friend, a partner, or someone we can trust. It doesn't always work that way. Even with beautiful relationships, they may not always be willing to come with you, and you'll have to decide whether it's worth it to you to go it alone.

You don't need to make it happen under thirty, forty, or fifty. You need something that lights you up because it holds meaning for you. It could be a posh business or pottery. It could be weight lifting or baking sourdough bread.

It could be career-oriented or simply art that you create for yourself.

It's the combination of the small things that we do in all areas of our lives that leads to a feeling of purpose. A group of tiny commitments that fill our hearts and souls. I know it seems like that can't possibly be the case, but it is. It really is. And when we settle for big wins and validation for being cool, we miss this. I know we're old enough to know this, and yet it still comes up, no matter your age. When we allow other people's projections to stop us, we miss this. But there comes a moment when we take that brave step to change direction. We realize we're done pretending it's all okay, and done letting ourselves down. We've hit our rock bottom.

When this happens, everything shifts.

Rock bottom is different for everyone, and I used to dislike this term until I realized how much of a gift it can be to recognize that you're done with carrying on with life as is. The negative connotation that one must endure so much harm before making a change felt like a self-fulfilling prophecy; I didn't want to say it out loud to myself, nor to any of my clients. *You'll know you're ready for change when everything in your life feels unbearable and you can't continue that way any longer;* that's not the type of affirmation I'd put on a T-shirt.

But this is part of it, whether I like it or not. For many, rock bottom doesn't have to be an extreme scenario. It can be the frozen smiles we place on our faces to hide our pain. It can be waking up each day with nothing to look forward to and no idea where to go from there. It can be realizing your relationships are a combination of people you love dearly, but around whom you've never felt comfortable being your real self. It can be realizing you have a deep purpose, a way you'd like your life to feel, that you haven't given to yourself, and you're scared because what if you never do.

Rock bottom could be realizing you're wearing a mask in the first place.

That mask you thought you were wearing for yourself was a mask you wore for everyone else, and it only hurt you. Every single time you put it on, it felt like the only way people would notice you, and it hurts. That's the feeling of being an imposter. That's why you thought you didn't belong. But even if people asked you to do what made them feel comfortable, it never meant that you had to. It doesn't mean that you need to continue.

Many people will realize that their rock bottom was riding the same train, day after day, year after year, allowing those same harmful messages to become ingrained within them as truths. We all encounter areas of doubt in our lives. You can be confident and still struggle with something that someone else finds easy. This is why comparisons limit us, because we don't know others' truth.

> **Blank Slate Energy**
>
> Ask yourself, when did you hit your rock bottom? How can you transmute that low into the moment you decide to bet on yourself again?

The Seven C that rings most true here is **choice**. You may have never felt the freedom to choose what you want for yourself because Little You felt limited by what you *had* to do for others. To pretend our circumstances are easy ignores the reality many of us face as parents, caretakers, and adults with responsibilities that feel heavy, time-consuming, and sometimes unfair.

Remembering the places where you <u>do</u> have a choice is essential. There are so many things we tell ourselves we must do that we don't have to. Remember, you're allowed to say no, even if you've only ever experienced being validated through giving, nurturing, and caring for others. Now that you've gotten on this new train, ready to say yes to a new path, where will you go, and are you willing to do it as you?

Are you willing to walk into rooms where you don't know anyone, but still go because you know you have to be there? Because you choose to? Are you willing to say yes to opportunities that have always felt too scary, too big, too much? Are you finally ready to stop talking about *what you've always wanted to do* and instead **choose** to do it? Are you ready to start living for you?

If you're not intentional about what you choose, you'll replace all the harmful train stops mentioned previously with new ones that don't sound as harsh but are still roadblocks. Imposter Station becomes *Maybe When I'm Older Lane. Who Do You Think You Are Street* becomes *I Can't Find the Time Street.* And *It'll Never Happen for You* becomes the dreaded *If It's Meant to Be, It'll Be.*

"If It's Meant to Be, It'll Be" is, in my opinion, the biggest killer of dreams. People put their faith in things happening on their behalf, without remembering that they have to make a choice. You must choose it. You must take steps. You must move toward it. You need to put in effort to make this happen. Even if it falls right into your lap, you still must choose.

You may not see this as a mask we wear, but it is. Our

masks aren't just those we wear for other people's comfort; our masks are also beliefs we hold that keep us hidden from our dreams.

It's time to say yes to passing through new stations. *I Belong at This Table Street. I Am Bigger Than You Could Ever Imagine Road.* And *I Will Thrive Lane.* We are done pretending for their comfort. Live your gifts out loud. Humble for who, and where? Why? Don't be afraid of being boastful. Overdo it. Go for it. It's time to leave the fear of standing in your greatness behind and own this space. We've been waiting for you to arrive.

Come Back to Yourself

While you're getting ready in the morning, look in the mirror and share three things that you're proud of yourself for doing. These three things could've occurred at any time in your life. Recite these three things each time you look in the mirror today, or share new things if they come to mind. The point is to look yourself in the eyes and BOAST.

You deserve this celebration. You've worked hard; you've earned it.

Now it's time to fully walk in what belongs to you.

in this era . . .
you're softer than you've ever been
happier than you've ever been
wiser than you've ever been
in this era,
you are free

15 Will You Accept the Invitation?

If art imitates life, I hope you dream in color.

I hope that you allow your life to be a reflection of what's possible when you refuse to believe your past is the only place where rebirth happens. I hope your life is a mirror for what happens when you say yes to blooming in a new season. A new era. Your comeback era.

My art often imitates my life, and the lives of those who live close to me, so it shouldn't have been a surprise when my husband received the opportunity to do something different in his career that would check all the Seven C's when I was writing this book. Something that he never would've considered before diving into purpose with me and, most importantly, with himself. This new opportunity would also give him time back, which meant he'd have the freedom to choose some of the things he's always wanted, that he didn't feel he had time for. But this opportunity didn't arrive as a gift with a bow. It came like a nightmare.

This new beginning was his pre-regret phase, where nothing had failed yet and nothing was wrong *yet*. And still, when we receive invitations for something new, perhaps before we're ready, it doesn't feel good. It feels alarming watching everything turned upside down.

Although I don't know what the future holds and how his purpose will unfold as he continues to grow, I know that this small step of allowing himself to **want more** while going for it has changed his life. I interviewed him for this book, although I later decided the conversation and breakthrough that he/we had was truly only for us to witness, but know this:

The realizations, understandings, and memories you've had while reading this book are genuine.

We live in a world where content is constantly curated to inspire us, and we've become so accustomed to consuming twenty-second videos and moving on to the next thing, we've lost the ability to engage in the deep and meaningful work of integration, even when we're deeply moved. These deeply feeling moments are special, primarily when we act on them. These awakenings are extraordinary, especially when we use them to move us forward. Your remembering is special, and not because it's rare, but because you feel safe enough to witness yourself.

I asked each person I interviewed the same questions you asked yourself at the beginning of each chapter. I had the beautiful experience of watching their facial expressions every single time the question landed with them. I saw as their minds immediately trailed back to a specific time, place, or belief that led them to answer each question in their unique way.

As each person shared their story, they experienced realizations and awakenings as they spoke it out loud. There's something incredibly special about speaking your truth out loud and having your experience witnessed. When my husband and I heard him say out loud, *I could do this job for the next thirty years for us,* we couldn't hide from the reality of his situation anymore. We couldn't pretend that this was something he was happy doing. We couldn't pretend that this sacrifice he was making was worth it or necessary. And although we're so grateful for what we have, we're also aware that not being able to do what he wanted would be devastating to him.

When you admit those kinds of truths out loud or on the page, it shifts something in you and in the people you care about. What matters to you is highlighted in your mind. What no longer matters, or never mattered, is clarified. You must adjust.

With that in mind, I present to you these final invitations. The first is an invitation to come back to you, an invitation to **your comeback era.** The era that Little You has been waiting for, for a long time. To love and to cherish yourself. To honor the paths you've walked before and the dreams you've held for far too long. Do you accept the invitation to dream again, unlocking anything that's been wanting to come free in your life? Do you accept the invitation to say what you want out loud, being a disrupter to the system of silence that so many of us have pledged allegiance to for far too long?

Do you accept the invitation to say what you want with your whole chest? No longer holding back because you think it's what will keep the peace, but fully committing to find peace in what is true to you? Do you accept the invitation to walk away when you need to? Never using endings as ultimatums but knowing exactly when you've overstayed your welcome in a relationship, experience, or time?

Do you accept the invitation to create? To allow the world around you to inspire you, even if the inspiration isn't shiny and bright? To find a way to hold both the joy of creating and the pain of creation at the same time?

Do you accept that these invitations will never force you to make a decision? If you ignore their knock, they will honor you and go quiet, because it's your life. But they won't give up on you; they'll sneak in at night, waking you to try and get your attention in any way they can.

Do you accept these invitations will sometimes arrive when you're covered in grief, when the last thing that you want is to do anything? That you could've just survived the most insurmountable loss, and there's an invitation waiting until you have the strength to say yes? Grief can harden our hearts, but there's a window where grief makes you so pliable, so soft, you become a living mold of what you've always wanted. Grief makes time and reality so vivid, and it's undeniable that loss, mortality, and endings of all kinds are part of life. Do you accept that even in your darkest hours, these invitations will come if they need to, trying to catch you in this pliable moment when you've slowed down enough to listen and you're soft enough to be moved?

A powerful thing happens when you finally say *yes*. God, the Universe, whatever you believe, begins to act on your behalf. The person who recommends the book you need while you stand in line at your coffee shop, which you visit every day. You've never seen them before, and you never see them again. The friendship that's been draining you ends without the brutal ending you were preparing for—it's easy and light. Things begin to fall into place as a *thank-you* from the cosmos because you've said yes. It sounds mystical, it sounds out there, but it's not. I'm sure you've experienced those moments when, because you followed your gut or your truth, it all begins to happen for you.

Remember, this is your life. Your season. Your era.
Your purpose is your guiding light.

It won't lead you to places of harm.
It won't put you in situations you're not equipped for.
You won't always feel this way, because living in
  alignment takes guts.
So much courage.
It's hard, no other way to explain it.
But it will keep you from feeling as if you're only here
  to waste away.
You're not here to serve others, but never yourself.
Your purpose will give you a life where people show
  up for you.

Your purpose is an invitation from your soul.

This invitation comes from the deepest, realist, purest part of you. We know it doesn't only have to do with money, validation, fame, or any of the things attributed to a false sense of self-discovery. Yes, you can be in your purpose and have all those things. But you could also be in your purpose and have none of those things.

Your soul is calling you back to yourself. I've always believed that when we're born, we're as close to God as we can be. That we hold answers to ourselves, the Universe, and others. That we speak "soul" as a language, and that's why children tell an unapologetic truth. We say children have no filter, but the truth should be unfiltered. What children haven't learned is we live in a world where the truth is left behind. Children haven't learned how to deliver the truth with kindness because they haven't learned that the truth can be hurtful. The gift of growing up is we can tap into the truth but deliver it with kindness.

Your soul is calling you back to a version of you before you forgot the truth. Little You only ignored your discernment to protect you; and although you let it go, those ingrained guides have never forgotten you. When you say yes, even when it's hard, you're reunited.

You've traveled from Curiosity to Comeback

By saying yes to living in your purpose, you've also said yes to releasing the guilt, shame, and barriers that blocked you in the past. I know some of those old feelings might creep up at what feels like the worst possible moment, but you have what it takes to face them now. You have the tools, and this was always the goal.

So, please take a moment to honor how far you've come.

In Part I: Curiosity, you bravely asked yourself the questions that matter. You reconnected with Little You, bringing kindness and compassion into your internal conversations. You acknowledged that you know what you want and how tough it can be to give it to yourself. Most importantly, you identified the parts of yourself that were left behind.

This is BIG work. Please don't take it lightly. Celebrate yourself.

Then . . .

In Part II: Remembering, you reclaimed and remembered the parts of yourself that were left behind, bringing along any parts you want to keep close. You recognized that rinse-and-repeat cycles have kept you stuck and considered what it might take to start again. And bravely, you remembered—the good and the challenging. You explored the Seven C's, solidifying what you need to bring purpose into your everyday life.

Round of applause. This is the part so many won't do because it's tough to remember. If you don't do part two, it's hard to get to part three. But you did it.

Lastly . . .

In Part III: Blank Slate Energy, you acknowledged you're in a pre-regret state, the space before any future mistakes. You're no longer allowing the past to keep you stuck; you're looking forward. You are grounded in the *present,* embracing a life without pretending, a life where you get to be your whole self.

And now you're ready to take it a step further and accept this invitation to your comeback era—a reunion with you.

We've talked about the Seven C's, but you haven't had an opportunity to explore the way you approach each of them in your own life. I placed this in the last chapter because you've learned so much about being compassionately honest with yourself and how it truly benefits you. You now have all the tools you need to approach this assessment with kindness while continuing to grow.

Think of this as your road map, designed to help you live your purpose and expand where you're ready. No judgments allowed here! Okay?

For each C below, you'll rate yourself on a scale of 1–5 on each question. After you finish answering the questions, for each section, you'll add the two numbers together for each C. For example, if you scored 2 for question one and 4 for question two under the Commitment section, you would add them together to get a total score of 6 for Commitment. At the end, you'll use the **Gain Curiosity** sheet, not to judge but to get curious about where you land in each area. This is information to help you heal, learn, grow, and repeat. And we'll do this a million times, if we're lucky. Feel free to take this assessment anytime you need clarity about where your energy is going, anytime things start to feel stagnant, or if you want some blank slate energy.

YOUR COMEBACK ERA ROAD MAP

Quick Reminder: On the scale of 1–5, 1 means you struggle with it and 5 means you're excelling at it.

Commitment

When I commit to doing something meaningful for myself, I follow through on it. Circle one:

1 2 3 4 5

My yes is intentional, and I show up for myself regularly. Circle one:

1 2 3 4 5

Community

I ask for help and allow my community to be there for me. Circle one:

1 2 3 4 5

I know vulnerability is a strength, and I often lean in to it.
Circle one:

1   2   3   4   5

Creativity

I don't put pressure on myself to be an expert in order to
create. Circle one:

1   2   3   4   5

I can think of an area I regularly use as a creative outlet.
Circle one:

1   2   3   4   5

Compelling

I'm inspired and excited by the things in my life, especially
areas where I can make a positive impact. Circle one:

1   2   3   4   5

My yes comes with boundaries. I choose the things that fill
me. Circle one:

1   2   3   4   5

Confirming

I can feel in my body when I've said yes to something that's
for me. Circle one:

1   2   3   4   5

I spend my time in places that feel good and that reflect
what I want in life. Circle one:

1   2   3   4   5

Choice

I spend my time how I'd like instead of how others believe I should. Circle one:

1   2   3   4   5

I'm willing to pivot when things don't go as I had hoped. Circle one:

1   2   3   4   5

Challenging

I know that healthy growth opportunities stretch my capabilities, and I seek them out. Circle one:

1   2   3   4   5

I look forward to learning new things and try to do this often. Circle one:

1   2   3   4   5

GAIN CURIOSITY

8–10 points: Your Comeback Era

- This C is a current strength of yours; lean in to it. Let this C guide and support you in bravely making small steps. This is the area where you excel; continue to shine brightly. With this C, you are in blank slate energy, ready to take off. Go for it.

- **Use this to your advantage:** Use this C to make your significant steps, big moves, and big changes because this is an area where you thrive! Even if things go awry, you'll be able to pick up right where you left off.

5–7 points: Remembering

- This C shows you've been taking risks, and it's paying off! I see you've been practicing, putting yourself out there, and pivoting when needed. C's that show up here are usually evidence of you working to build a muscle in a place that requires some growth, and that's amazing! With this C, you may still be trying to remember who you are. This is brave work you've done! Celebrate yourself!

- **Use this to your advantage:** This C is a place where you can practice being brave. Instead of taking a small step, in this area, you could take a small leap. Send the email, ask for help, and draft the story, even if you're not ready to publish. You're getting stronger here, so you don't want to put too much weight on these C's, but they're prepared to grow!

2–4 points: Get Curious

- This C is where the magic happens, where you set up your vision. What will your life look like when you're able to lean in here? This is for those small steps. And know that every C that you excel in above was once right here. We all start somewhere. More than anything, this area right here needs your **curiosity**, not your judgment. What do you need to take the next small step? Remember all the ways you're already showing up. You're doing the work, love.

- **Possible Small Steps to Expand:** Watch a show or video about painting instead of doing the painting. Write a

Post-it reminder and let that be the end; no need to follow through yet. Take a different block home. Try hot sauce. Buy a vegetable you've never tried. Find ways to interrupt the patterns you have here, just like we talked about earlier. Expand; you're ready to move. Let's do this.

NOW THAT YOU UNDERSTAND YOUR CURRENT SITUATION and future direction, I've created invitations for each C so that you can start where you feel excited to begin. Remember, this is about what feels meaningful to you. You can choose all seven, but I encourage you to start with one or two. You can always come back and try something new. Pivoting is your best friend.

WILL YOU ACCEPT THIS INVITATION TO COMMIT?

If you're ready to commit, repeat after me:

I don't know where this journey will take me, but I trust I have what it takes to succeed. With my pockets full of wisdom, lessons, wins, and strengths, I bring all my excitement and fear too. I use it all for my good. I use it all to be who I'm meant to be.

I commit to showing up when it's hard. I commit to showing up when I'm unsure. I commit to showing up when no one else wants to come with me. I commit to showing up when I must start over. I commit to showing up as many times as needed because I'm committed to myself.

Next Small Step

For the next three days, please commit to one small commitment for five minutes.

For example, if you've decided to write, for the next three days, you'll write for five minutes. You can use a pen, computer, or use your phone. But for at least five minutes each day, you're going to write for three days.

Notice what you learn about yourself. Is it easier than you thought? Do you need more time? Is it hard to get started? Just get curious and remember, your job here isn't to write the final piece; it's to practice commitment.

What I know will happen: You'll start thinking about your ideas, struggles, excitement, or feelings of being overwhelmed about this commitment throughout your day. Whether the emotions are positive or challenging, guess what? You're still committed. Whether there's an easy fix or it's going to take time, guess what? You're still committing.

Sometimes we confuse commitment with perfection, and that's how we end up quitting. One thing goes wrong, and we don't want to face ourselves. Listen, the more pocket wisdom, the better! Just be sure to keep showing up!

You can continue after three days, or start exploring other commitments that matter to you.

WILL YOU ACCEPT THIS INVITATION TO LEAN IN TO COMMUNITY?

If you're ready to commit, repeat after me:

I'm ready to lean in to community, allowing the people around me to reflect the goodness that lives in me. I know when I find my people and trust that it's safe to lean in to them, it will change my life. I won't be doing this on my own anymore because I've let them in.

I commit to vulnerability, even when I want to hide. I

commit to asking for help, even when I would rather do it all alone. I commit to letting people see me at my best and in the moments when I need them to lift me. I commit to being seen, to being witnessed, to being loved, and to not just being the reliable one. I'm a full yes to community.

Next Small Step

I know there's something you could use a little help with. Maybe you've been wanting someone to join you at a cooking class. Maybe you've wanted to share some new ideas with a friend. Or perhaps you need someone to help you with your résumé, as you're looking for new jobs.

Today, I want you to ask two people for help. Choose something that feels like too much to ask, but is still a small request to the person you know well, someone who's already shown you they are there for you. Go ahead and ask.

Text the person (or call if you prefer) for something you need help with that's more practical than emotional. To be clear, you're asking for help with things you genuinely need assistance with and would usually figure out on your own. You won't make this decision based on how busy you think they are or how much you think it will be a burden. You're going to allow them to decide whether they have time to help you or how much help they can provide.

They may not be able to help you immediately. They may not be able to help at all. This doesn't mean you aren't loved, seen, or respected. This means you need to ask someone else. And we're not talking about people in your life who never show up; we're talking about the people you know, love, and trust. *Your people.* You know that if they can't, it's because they can't, and your work is not to make this a pattern of you keeping all your needs stuffed inside to manage alone. It's time for you to ask for help, especially since you give so freely. How do I know? The people who struggle with asking for help are often willing to help others. Always. It's time you allowed your needs to get met too.

Below, I've included a short script that you can use and adapt for your initial conversations. I will not let the fact that you don't know how to ask be a barrier to receiving support. We're in this together, my friend.

Script 1: Hey ______, how are you? I have a quick question; please answer when you have a moment. I know you're great at ______ and I'm trying to figure out ______, but I'm struggling with these next steps. Honestly, I'm on the verge of quitting/giving up/walking away (add your real emotions here and be vulnerable with the folks who love you so they can support you). When you have space, I'd love help with how I can do ______. Or, if you know of any resources or someone who can offer support, I'd truly appreciate it.

Script 2: Hey ______, how are you? I'm trying to ______ and have hit a roadblock. I've seen you do ______ and it feels similar to where I'm going, but I'm overwhelmed (or enter the emotion you feel comfortable sharing here). **Option 1:** If possible, I'd love some time to chat with you to understand more about ______. **Option 2:** If possible, can you help me build ______. **Option 3:** If possible, could you let me know if we could spend some time doing ______ together? I truly value your opinion and could really use the support. Appreciate you!

Tailor these in any way you see fit. I wanted to get you going. Let's do this!

WILL YOU ACCEPT THIS INVITATION TO CREATE?

If you're ready to commit, repeat after me:

I know I'm born to create. I've always seen my gifts, and I'm finally ready to tap into them. There are so many things I've wanted to try and now I'm making space. On the way home from work, while commuting, or when I have time with friends, I'm finding ways to integrate creativity into my life.

There's nothing I must do to be creative. Yes, there are things for me to learn, but I'm already creative. I commit to creating joy. I commit to creating outside of my job. I commit to creating in any small way that I can. I'm ready.

Next Small Step

Want to write? Carry a small notebook and pen or use your phone, and begin. Start with nothing to say, start with the dream you had last night. Set a timer for five minutes and go.

Want to paint? Head to the dollar store and grab the first set of paints that catches your interest. Spend no more than five bucks and go. Get the kid's painting kit or the blank canvas and go for it. Set a timer for five minutes and let it all go.

Want to show your creativity through your clothes? Start with your shoes. Find a unique way to switch up your outfit by making a subtle change during the last step of your routine. It's easier than figuring out how to change everything at the beginning, and it's a small way to see what you like. When you change your shoes, you'll notice the bag that would look nice with them. Or, you'll try a different coat with those shoes.

It's time to start. No matter what it is you'd like to do creatively, give yourself the chance. Five minutes or less in the beginning. Start small!

WILL YOU ACCEPT THIS INVITATION TO HAVE A COMPELLING LIFE?

If you're ready to commit, repeat after me:

I'm ready to lean in to my life and fill it with things that inspire me. I won't only choose what feels safe or what I think is the right thing to do in the world. I will choose what feels right for me.

I commit to pivoting when boredom pops up. I commit to staying curious about my routines and incorporating new ideas, keeping things fresh for myself. I commit to allowing life to lead me down paths that interest me, even if it's the opposite of what I do for a living or what I'm known for. I commit to being a curious human who's ready to explore.

Next Small Step

What creative thing did you choose in the last small step? If you didn't pick anything, what creative thing is calling you right now? Gardening? Cooking?

I want you to find a class. Bring a friend or go solo, whichever feels most comfortable. If a class isn't accessible to you, invite friends to a get-together and have your own "class" together.

Community sparks inspiration. Participating in community activities stretches you. Expand, love.

Oh, and don't just say *yeah, that's a great idea.*

Take five minutes and research some classes in your area. If those don't work, send a text to your group chat and ask if you can get together and do the things. Use the script I created if you need help. You've got this!

WILL YOU ACCEPT THIS INVITATION OF CHOICE?

If you're ready to commit, repeat after me:

I'm ready to choose myself. I'll come back to this place as many times as needed, because I know that sometimes we forget to stand in our power. When I've forgotten to stand in my power, I'll reclaim what I am and what I've always known.

That I can choose.

And I commit to choosing my life. I commit to sharing my dreams with my partner, my kids, my friends, and my family, and to choosing to live out loud. I commit to staying grounded in my choices, even if it scares others. I love myself too much to limit the many talents and strengths that are within me.

Next Small Step

Put this affirmation on your mirror right where you can see it each day:

I love myself too much to let other people dictate the life I live. I decide. Me.

WILL YOU ACCEPT THIS INVITATION, EVEN THOUGH IT WILL BE CHALLENGING?

If you're ready to commit, repeat after me:

To commit even though it will be challenging is a s. t. r. e. t. c. h. I used to think, *I've had enough challenges in my life,* so I only sought out what felt easy and fun. But I'm strong when it comes to drama, trauma, and rising again.

I'm innovative, a problem solver, and I have a unique perspective on life and the world that enables me to take on healthy challenges and thrive. I commit to saying yes to challenges, such as embracing new things that scare me, asking for help, and allowing people in my community to be there for me. I commit to learning a new creative way of being, no matter how challenging it may be at first. I commit to the challenge of allowing inspiration to lead me, a constant guide toward new doors opening. I commit to choosing myself, no matter how challenging this may be for my relationships, my job, and areas of my life that have expected me to shrink. I commit to standing tall.

I accept these invitations, one of the biggest challenges I've ever said yes to.

But I wholeheartedly choose myself.

Next Small Step

Now that you've accepted your invitation(s), I invite you to clarify your focus as much as possible. Are you learning to bake? Are you looking for a new job? Are you working on communication in your marriage? Are you ready to start dating? Are you picking up painting again? Are you going on a health journey? Remember, having a meaningful life isn't about finding *the thing;* it's about having a life that reflects you, the whole you. This is living in your purpose.

You're starting with one small change, one small addition, one small moment that you know will feel so good, so electrifying, and that has been calling to you. It could be as simple as cleaning out one drawer in the bathroom or finally buying a trash can that matches your decor! Start small and keep going by using the following:

I accept this invitation, and . . .
I'm committing to ________.
My community will help me ________.
I'm creating ________ and it's compelling to me because
________.
I choose me.
I also choose ________.
There will be challenges. I've already experienced
________.
Here's what I also know to be true about me. I always
________.

Here's an example of what that could look like:

I accept this invitation, and . . .
I'm committing to <u>trying a new style</u>.
My community will help me <u>by voting on looks I text over for advice</u>.
I'm creating <u>a new way of seeing myself</u> and it's compelling to me because <u>I want to change my relationship with my body</u>.
I choose me.
I also choose <u>variety and fresh energy in my attire</u>.
There will be challenges. I've already experienced <u>spending hours trying to find something that fits me the way I want it to and feeling defeated</u>.

Here's what I also know to be true about me. I
always <u>get back up and try again. Even if I quit, it's</u>
<u>momentary. The little things can be important too.</u>

Before you're officially off on your journey, I have one
last thing to share. And do this only when you're ready,
only when it feels exciting to do. Because you're crafting
your future, using your vision to speak life into what you
want to come true. I want you to bring your best energy to
this, because we are powerful and we want you standing in
your power, speaking beautiful words over your future and
your life.

I invite you to write a letter as if it's from you in the future.
Remember, you are living in your future's past.

Future You will use this letter to tell current you all the
things they're so proud you chose for yourself. Let this letter
be a manifesting reminder of your why. You are doing this
work because of the meaning it brings you and how it will
change your life now and forever.

What's *Future You* going to say about Their Past?

Imagine your future self is reflecting on the beautiful
things you've done over the past year. Why will your future
self be thanking you? What has changed in your beliefs? How
is your life different? Please write it down.

Bonus: Take it a step further and write letters from your
future self five years from now, ten years from now, and
beyond. Have fun with it. Get unserious. Dream.

I leave you with this invitation toward curiosity, which will
undoubtedly guide you toward remembering who you are
and how you want to spend your life. You can talk about what

you want to do all day, but until you take a step toward it, it remains just a dream. You make it real through movement. Many of us are stuck because we spend our time talking not only about what we feel we've missed, but also about others and what we believe they're missing.

You don't have time for this. Not because time is running out, but because your gifts are waiting for you, and they've been waiting a long time. Don't let those distractions block you from living in your blessings. They're on the other side of this moment; step through it.

Little You will help you remember that this life you're living right now is a privilege. Each day you get to do it again is a gift. Each moment you remember is a gift. Each time you say yes is a gift. And Little You won't remind you through long boring lessons of how ungrateful you've been, or through nagging you to *get it together*. Those internal voices aren't Little You.

Little You reminds you by loving you and making you feel worth it when it feels like you're not. Take this love in. When it arrives through Little You or the people in your life, allow yourself to be cared for and held.

Every yes you speak, even if you whisper it, syncs you up to your purpose. Every yes you speak only asks that you be willing. Every yes you speak will help you extinguish the negative thoughts that say the way it was is the way it will always be. It wasn't true then and it isn't true now.

If art imitates life, I hope you make it magical. I hope you take the things you once called "weird" and put them on display for all to see. I hope your past begins to feel far away, so you can't remember how you could've denied you for so long. And with love, I hope you answer exactly why you denied you for so long so that you never forget and never let it happen again.

If you do forget, as we often do, I hope you know Little You will be there waiting with open arms, ready to guide you back to you. Never taking for granted how hard the path you walk is, and only there as a loving friend and companion. Ready to usher in a new season, a new invitation, a new world.

As it always has been. Walk into it. The Comeback Era.

Acknowledgments

Thank you to God, my ancestors, and all the angels that conspired on my behalf to help me through this book while life was really throwing everything my way. I'm grateful for favor, IYKYK.

I'm so grateful to my team: Kim, Kari, Angela, HarperOne, CAA, and all the folks who are helping me bring this to life. Wow, a third book!

Thanks to my husband for listening to me go on and on about this topic for two years and encouraging me to start the book even though I was in the middle of my second book's tour. I don't know how you deal with all my ideas lolol.

Lia, Amanda, Britt, Deesha, and Chloe, thank you SO MUCH for trusting me to tell your stories in this book. You're each an inspiration and I can't wait to hear others talk about how much your perseverance has resonated and helped them.

And thank you to all my friends who have supported, guided, or lent a hand during this book process. You're all just as busy as me and yet you take the time to show up for me, and believe me, I won't forget it. Thank you!

All the folks who have been following me since *The Sugar Jar* days, thank you! I hope this book helps you continue the work! We've got this! xx

I met Lia while on a trip to Costa Rica, traveling from the airport on a two-and-a-half-hour car ride to our resort. We used that bumpy ride to jump into a friendship that feels like we've known each other for lifetimes. She is such a kind person, and one of the most thoughtful people I've ever met. She is naturally inquisitive, which is probably one of her greatest gifts as a therapist. You feel like she wants to know you, and that presence alone is healing.

She also cares deeply about the world around her and is an activist, writer, and podcaster.

You can find her work on her Instagram and website: @ lialoveavellino, linktr.ee/lialoveavellino.

Amanda and I had a similar experience, meeting a few years ago through work. Within five minutes of meeting, we were synced up, helping someone figure out what *sign* they were getting from the Universe after they shared that glass kept breaking around them. We just tuned in immediately. She's the kind of person you can't shock and can tell anything to. And she is hilarious.

She's a phenomenal businessperson who has fully pivoted into spirituality, building an uplifting community that helps to replace overwhelm and chaos with calm and safety.

You can find her work on her Instagram and website: @ amandabaudier, linktr.ee/amandabaudier.

Britt is one of the most honest people I've ever met. She will say what she's thinking and it will often be the thing a lot of people are thinking but will never say. She's caring and unbelievably smart. And one of the kindest and most loyal folks around. When I went to her book tour in her hometown, I saw her shine in her circus greatness, as she booked a class for all of us to attend. She is one of the bravest people I know because the hardest thing we can do is say yes to what we want in spite of others.

Britt is a licensed neuro psychotherapist, author, and speaker, and her interview blew me away. She could've easily neuro scienced me down, but instead she shared her human experience in the most thoughtful way, which I'm so grateful for. I'm so lucky I got to share her beautiful story in this book.

You can find her work on her Instagram and website: @ brittfrank, brittfrank.com.

Deesha is the former social secretary for the Obama administration. The literal woman behind bringing culture, specifically Black culture, into the White House for the first time, Deesha took the opportunity she was given and brought her dreams (and ours) to life.

She is one of the most giving people I've ever met, always available, always supporting, and always thinking about you. She finds time for you when no one else with her schedule would. I would imagine almost everyone in Deesha's life thinks they are the most important thing on her list, because that's how she treats you. She is gold.

You can find her work on her Instagram and website: @ deedyer267, deeshadyer.com.

Chloe is so many beautiful things. She is a storyteller, she is a painter, she is a writer. When you look up "artist" and "curator" in the dictionary, her face and name should be alongside. She is the most beautiful connector, always thinking of how two people who don't know each other absolutely need to meet to make the world and their lives genuinely better.

I've dined on the best food sitting on cushions in her dining and living room, laughing among wine and friends. If I had to describe Chloe's essence, it would be home. She is a brilliant writer who hosts writing salons all over—from DC to Arizona to Greece—while also working for the Gates Foundation doing some of the most amazing work in Africa and throughout the world.

You can find her work on her Instagram and website: @ chloe_dulce, linktr.ee/chloelouvouezo.

Notes

Chapter 1: What Did Little You Always Know Was True?

1. Doris Baumann and Willibald Ruch, "What Constitutes a Fulfilled Life? A Mixed Methods Study on Lay Perspectives Across the Lifespan," *Frontiers in Psychology*, September 29, 2022, https://doi.org/10.3389/fpsyg.2022.982782.

Chapter 2: What If I Don't Have Enough Time?

1. Centers for Disease Control and Prevention, "Life Expectancy," FastStats, National Center for Health Statistics, June 5, 2025, https://www.cdc.gov/nchs/fastats/life-expectancy.htm.

2. Jesús Montero-Marín and Javier García-Campayo, "A Newer and Broader Definition of Burnout: Validation of the 'Burnout Clinical Subtype Questionnaire (BCSQ-36),'" *BMC Public Health*, 2010, https://doi.org/10.1186/1471-2458-10-302.

3. Evangelia Demerouti, Arnold B. Bakker, and Wilmar B. Schaufeli, "Spillover and Crossover of Exhaustion and Life Satisfaction among Dual-Earner Parents," *Journal of Vocational Behavior* 67, no. 2 (2005): 266–89, https://doi.org/10.1016/j.jvb.2004.07.001.

Chapter 4: What If I'm the Reason I'm Unhappy?

1. R. E. Beaty, M. Benedek, P. J. Silvia, and D. L. Schacter, "Creativity and the Default Network: A Functional Connectivity Analysis of the Creative Brain at Rest." *Proceedings of the National Academy of Sciences* 111, no. 10 (2014): 4004–4009, https://doi.org/10.1016/j.neuropsychologia.2014.09.019; L. Shalev, A. R. Hariri, et al., "Cumulative Risk on Oxytocin-Pathway Genes Impairs Default Mode Network Connectivity in Trauma-Exposed Youth," *Frontiers in Endocrinology* 11 no. 335 (2020), https://doi.org/10.3389/fendo.2020.00335.

Chapter 7: What Did Little You Want to Be When You Grew Up?

1. R. A. Stebbins, *Serious Leisure: A Perspective for Our Time* (Transaction Publishers, 2007); R. A. Stebbins, "The Serious Leisure Perspective: a Critical Review," *Leisure Studies* 37, no. 4 (2018): 429–42, www.researchgate.net/publication/304856764_The_Serious_Leisure_Perspective; Y. Mansourian, "From Serious Leisure to Passionate Pastime: Expanding the Conceptual Landscape, *Leisure Studies* 43, no. 2 (2024): 158-74, https://doi.org/10.1080/02614367.2024.2413055.

Chapter 8: Do You Want What You've Worked For?

1. T. Ben-Shahar, *Happier: Learn the Secrets to Daily Joy and Lasting Fulfillment* (McGraw-Hill, 2007).
2. S. L. Di Domenico and R. M. Ryan, "The Emerging Neuroscience of Intrinsic Motivation: A New Frontier in Self-Determination Research," *Frontiers in Human Neuroscience* 11, no. 145 (2017), https://www.frontiersin.org/articles/10.3389/fnhum.2017.00145/full; R. M. Ryan and E. L. Deci, "Intrinsic and Extrinsic Motivations: Classic Definitions and New Directions," *Contemporary Educational Psychology* 25, no. 1 (2000): 54–67. https://doi.org/10.1006/ceps.1999.1020.

References

American College of Obstetricians and Gynecologists. "Committee Opinion No.565: Hormone Therapy and Heart Disease." *Obstetrics and Gynecology* 121, no. 6 (2013): 1407–10. https://doi.org/10.1097/01.AOG0000431057.65953.5f.

Ashkenazi, M. *Handbook of Japanese Mythology.* ABC-CLIO, 2003.

Beaty, R. E., Benedek, M., Silvia, P. J., and Schacter, D. L. "Creativity and the Default Network: A Functional Connectivity Analysis of the Creative Brain at Rest." *Proceedings of the National Academy of Sciences* 111, no. 10 (2014): 4004–4009. https://doi.org/10.1073/pnas.1308310111.

Ben-Shahar, T. *Happier: Learn the Secrets to Daily Joy and Lasting Fulfillment.* McGraw-Hill, 2007.

Centers for Disease Control and Prevention. *"Life Expectancy."* National Center for Health Statistics, 2025. https://www.cdc.gov/nchs/fastats/life-expectancy.htm.

Demerouti, E., Bakkar, A. B., and Schaufeli, W. B. "Spillover and Crossover of Exhaustion and Life Satisfaction among Dual-Earner Parents," *Journal of Vocational Behavior* 67, no. 2 (2005): 266–89. https://doi.org/10.1016/j.jvb.2004.07.001.

Di Domenico, S. I., and Ryan, R. M. "The Emerging Neuroscience of Intrinsic Motivation: A New Frontier in Self-Determination Research" *Frontiers in Human Neuroscience* 11 (2017): 145. https://www.frontiersin.org/articles/10.3389/fnhum.2017.00145/full.

Hennessey, B. A., and Amabile, T. M. "Creativity." *Annual Review of Psychology* 61 (2010): 569–98. https://doi.org/10.1146/annurev.psych.093008.100416.

The Holy Bible: New International Version. Zondervan, 2011.

Jewish Publication Society. *Tanakh: The Holy Scriptures.* Jewish Publication Society, 1985.

Keri, A. "Blending Oxytocin and Dopamine with Everyday Creativity."

Scientific Reports 11, no. 1 (2021): 18204. https://doi.org/10.1038/s41598-021-95724-x.

Liu, Y., You, Y., Shan, J., and Lou, Y. "The Influence of Mindfulness on Mental Health: The Meditating Role of Social Connectedness and the Moderating Role of Emotion Regulation." *Frontiers in Psychology* 12, no. 795931 (2022). https://doi.org/10.3389/fpsyg.2021.795931.

Mansourian, Y. "From Serious Leisure to Passionate Pastime: Expanding the Conceptual Landscape." *Leisure Studies* 43, no. 2 (2024): 158–74. https://doi.org/10.1080/02614367.2024.2413055.

Montero-Marin, J., Garcia-Campayo, J., Demorouti, E., Salanova, M., and Bakker, A. B. "A Newer and Broader Definition of Burnout: Validation of the 'Burnout Clinical Subtype Questionnaire' (BCSQ-36)." *BMC Public Health* 10, no. 302 (2010). https://doi.org/10.1186/1471-2458-10-302.

Office for National Statistics. "National Life Tables-Life Expectancy in the UK: 2020 to 2022 (Statistical bulletin), 2024. https://www.ons.gov.uk/peoplepopulationandcommunity/birthsdeathsandmarriages/lifeexpectancies/bulletins/nationallifetablesunitedkingdom/2020to2022.

The Qur'an. Abdel Haleem, M.A.S., trans. Oxford University Press, 2008.

Rahula, W. *What the Buddha Taught.* Grove Press, 1974.

Ryan, R. M., and Deci, E. L. "Intrinsic and Extrinsic Motivations: Classic Definitions and New Directions." *Contemporary Educational Psychology* 25, no. 1 (2000): 54–67. https://doi.org/10.1006/ceps.1999.1020.

Shalev, I., Hariri, A. R., et al. "Cumulative Risk on Oxytocin-Pathway Genes Impairs Default Mode Network Connectivity in Trauma-Exposed Youth." *Frontiers in Endocrinology* 11, no. 335 (2020). https://doi.org/10.3389/fendo.2020.00335.

Stebbins, R. A. *Serious Leisure: A Perspective for Our Time.* Transaction Publishers, 2007.

Stebbins, R. A. "The Serious Leisure Perspective: A Critical Review." *Leisure Studies* 37, no. 4 (2018): 429–42. https://doi.org/10.1057/9781137399731_2.

Zimmer, H. *Myths and Symbols in Indian Art and Civilization.* Princeton University Press, 1946.